Competency Based Logbook for General Surgery and Allied Subjects

Name of the student ____

Name of the college ____

College roll number ____

Permanent address ____

Mobile number ____

Email ID ____

Competency Based Logbook for General Surgery and Allied Subjects

As per Competency Based Medical Education Curriculum (NMC)

Anurag Mishra MBBS MS DNB MNAMS FAIS FACS
Professor (Surgery)
Maulana Azad Medical College
Lok Nayak Hospital
New Delhi, India

Adiba Nizam MBBS MS DNB
Senior Resident
Maulana Azad Medical College
Lok Nayak Hospital
New Delhi, India

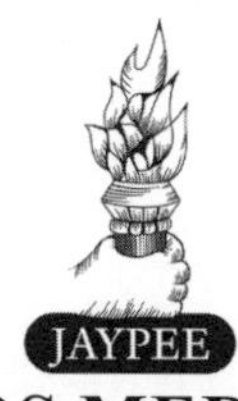

JAYPEE
JAYPEE BROTHERS MEDICAL PUBLISHERS
The Health Sciences Publisher
New Delhi | London

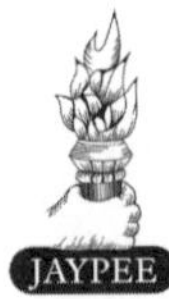 **Jaypee Brothers Medical Publishers (P) Ltd.**

Headquarters

Jaypee Brothers Medical Publishers (P) Ltd.
EMCA House
23/23-B, Ansari Road, Daryaganj
New Delhi - 110 002, India
Landline: +91-11-23272143, +91-11-23272703
+91-11-23282021, +91-11-23245672
Email: jaypee@jaypeebrothers.com

Corporate Office

Jaypee Brothers Medical Publishers (P) Ltd.
4838/24, Ansari Road, Daryaganj
New Delhi 110 002, India
Phone: +91-11-43574357
Fax: +91-11-43574314
Email: jaypee@jaypeebrothers.com

Overseas Office

J.P. Medical Ltd
83 Victoria Street, London
SW1H 0HW (UK)
Phone: +44 20 3170 8910
Fax: +44 (0)20 3008 6180
Email: info@jpmedpub.com

Website: www.jaypeebrothers.com
Website: www.jaypeedigital.com

Competency Based Logbook for General Surgery and Allied Subjects

First Edition: 2023

Reprint: 2024

ISBN: 978-93-5696-142-5

Printed at Sterling Graphics Pvt. Ltd.

Certificate

This is to certify that the candidate Ms/Mr _____________________, University enrolment number _____________________ admitted to _____________________________ College in the year ____________ has satisfactorily completed/has not completed all the assignments/requirements mentioned in the logbook of Surgery in the second professional, third professional part I and II years during the period from __________ to ________. She/he is eligible to appear for the summative university assessment as on the date mentioned below.

Signature of Faculty incharge

Countersignature by the Head of Department

(General Surgery)

Place:

Date:

Certificate

This is to certify that the candidate Ms/Mr ___________________, University enrolment number _________________ admitted to _________________________________ College in the year ___________ has satisfactorily completed/has not completed all the assignments/requirements mentioned in the logbook of Orthopedics in the second professional, third professional part I and II years during the period from _________ to ________. She/he is eligible to appear for the summative university assessment as on the date mentioned below.

Signature of Faculty incharge

Countersignature by the Head of Department

(Orthopedics)

Place:

Date:

Certificate

This is to certify that the candidate Ms/Mr _____________________, University enrolment number _________________ admitted to _________________________________ College in the year ____________ has satisfactorily completed/has not completed all the assignments/requirements mentioned in the logbook of Anesthesia in the second professional, third professional part I and II years during the period from __________ to _________. She/he is eligible to appear for the summative university assessment as on the date mentioned below.

Signature of Faculty incharge

Countersignature by the Head of Department

(Anesthesia)

Place:

Date:

Certificate

This is to certify that the candidate Ms/Mr ____________________, University enrolment number ____________________ admitted to ____________________ College in the year ___________ has satisfactorily completed/has not completed all the assignments/requirements mentioned in the logbook of Radiodiagnosis in the second professional, third professional part I and II years during the period from _________ to _______. She/he is eligible to appear for the summative university assessment as on the date mentioned below.

Signature of Faculty incharge

Countersignature by the Head of Department

(Radiodiagnosis)

Place:

Date:

Preface

A key aspect of the Competency based UG curriculum (2018) is emphasis on the acquisition of competencies for UG medical students in India. Completion of activities specified and submission of certified logbook is a prerequisite for a student to apply for summative examinations and graduation from the MBBS course.

'Logbook for General Surgery' aims to create a standard recording template for documenting the achievement of knowledge, skills, attitudes and selected competencies listed in the Competency based UG curriculum (2018) and the Regulations on Graduate Medical Education Part II (2019) for General Surgery and allied subjects including Anesthesia, Orthopedics and Radiology. AETCOM competencies have also been included in the logbook.

This logbook is designed according to the CBME guidelines as per the Revised National Medical Council Curriculum UG to provide an easy framework for students and educators for certifying achieved competencies and subcompetencies. We bring this first of a kind logbook in General Surgery which integrates recording certified achievement of competencies with academic presentations, achievements, publications, surgical procedures logbook, clinical cases logbook and more. This logbook has been compiled in a way that only one logbook will suffice for the General Surgery curriculum.

We hope that students find the first edition of the integrated logbook utilitarian and beneficial. Kindly reach out for suggestions for future editions.

Anurag Mishra
Adiba Nizam

Contents

Contents

General Instructions

1. The logbook is a record of the academic/co-curricular activities of the designated student, who would be responsible for maintaining his/her logbook.
2. The student is responsible for getting the entries in the logbook verified by the Faculty Incharge regularly.
3. Entries in the logbook will reflect the activities undertaken in the department and have to be scrutinized by the Head of the concerned department.
4. The logbook is a record of various activities by the student like:
   a. Overall participation and performance
   b. Attendance
   c. Participation in sessions
   d. Record of completion of pre-determined activities
   e. Acquisition of selected competencies.
5. The logbook is the record of work done by the candidate in that department/specialty and should be verified by the college before submitting the application of the students for the university examination.
6. A designated faculty member in each unit will coordinate and facilitate the activities of the learner, monitor progress, provide feedback and review the logbook/case record.
7. The logbook/case record must include the written case record prepared by the learner including relevant investigations, treatment and its rationale, hospital course, family and patient discussions, discharge summary, etc.
8. The logbook should also include records of outpatients assigned. Submission of the logbook/case record to the department is required for eligibility to appear for the final examination of the subject.

Explanation of each column in the logbook table

1	2	3	4	5	6	7	8
Competency	Name of Activity	Date completed (dd-mm-yyyy)	Attempt at activity First or Only (F) Repeat (R) Remedial (Re)	Rating Below (B) expectations Meets (M) expectations Exceeds (E) Expectations OR Numerical Score	Decision of Faculty Completed (C) Repeat (R) Remedial (Re)	Initial of Faculty and Date	Feedback Received Initial of Learner

1. The number of the competency addressed includes the subject initial and number (from Vol I, II, or III of the UG Curriculum), e.g., AN 2.1
2. Name of activity, e.g., Seminar on Liver or Group Discussion or Session 1 of CPR (if the institution has numbered each activity, the number may be entered)
3. Date the activity gets completed
4. Attempt at activity by learner: Indicate if:
   a. First attempt (or) only attempt
   b. Repeat (R) of a previously done activity
   c. Remedial activity (Re) based on the determination by the faculty

5. Rating—use one of three grades:
   a. Below expectations (B)
   b. Meets expectations (M)
   c. Exceeds expectations (E)
6. Decision of faculty
   a. C: Activity is completed, therefore closed and can be certified, if needed
   b. R: Activity needs to be repeated without any further intervention
   c. Re: Activity needs remedial action (usually done after repetition did not lead to satisfactory completion)
7. Initial (Signature) of faculty indicating the completion or other determination
8. Initial (Signature) of the learner if feedback has been received.

Logbook for General Surgery

"Goal—The aim of training in General Surgery is to impart such knowledge and skills that may enable him/her to diagnose and treat common surgical ailments. He/she shall have ability to diagnose and suspect with reasonable accuracy all acute and chronic surgical illnesses."

A key aspect of the new Competency-based UG Curriculum for Indian Medical Graduates is the emphasis on acquisition of competencies as a requisite for progression in the course. Active learning process by the student and his/her progression to achievement of competencies/predetermined tasks need to be documented. A record of activities completed and competencies acquired is necessary to ensure that the learner has acquired the key competencies. This logbook forms an integral part of the formative/continuous assessment program.

For satisfactory assessment in general surgery, the student must demonstrate:
1. Understanding of the structural and functional basis, principles of diagnosis and management of common surgical problems in adults and children
2. Ability to choose, calculate and administer appropriately intravenous fluids, electrolytes, blood and blood products based on the clinical condition
3. Ability to apply the principles of asepsis, sterilization, disinfection, rational use of prophylaxis, therapeutic utilities of antibiotics and universal precautions in surgical practice
4. Knowledge of common malignancies in India and their prevention, early detection and therapy
5. Ability to perform common diagnostic and surgical procedures at the primary care level
6. Ability to recognize, resuscitate, stabilize, and provide basic and advanced life support to patients following trauma
7. Ability to administer informed consent and counsel patient prior to surgical procedures
8. Commitment to advancement of quality and patient safety in surgical practice.
   The competencies prescribed by the erstwhile Medical Council of India in 2018 divide general surgery into 30 topics. The competencies to be sought at the end of undergraduate training are in the competency table on the next page.

Competency Table

GENERAL SURGERY

Number	Competency: The student should be able to	Domain K/S/A/C	Level K/KH/ SH/P	Core (Y/N)	Suggested Teaching Learning method	Suggested Assessment method	Number required to certify P
Topic: Metabolic Response to Injury Number of competencies: (03)					**Number of procedures that require certification: (NIL)**		
SU1.1	Describe basic concepts of homeostasis, enumerate the metabolic changes in injury and their mediators.	K	KH	Y	Lecture, Bedside clinic, Small group discussion	Written/Viva voce	
SU1.2	Describe the factors that affect the metabolic response to injury.	K	KH	Y	Lecture, Bedside clinic, Small group discussion	Written/Viva voce	
SU1.3	Describe basic concepts of perioperative care.	K	KH	Y	Lecture, Bedside clinic, Small group discussion	Written/Viva voce	
Topic: Shock Number of competencies: (03)					**Number of procedures that require certification: (NIL)**		
SU2.1	Describe pathophysiology of shock, types of shock and principles of resuscitation including fluid replacement and monitoring.	K	KH	Y	Lecture, Small group discussion	Written/Viva voce	
SU2.2	Describe the clinical features of shock and its appropriate treatment.	K	KH	Y	Lecture, Small group discussion	Written/Viva voce	
SU2.3	Communicate and counsel patients and families about the treatment and prognosis of shock demonstrating empathy and care	A/C	SH	Y	DOAP session	Skill assessment	
Topic: Blood and Blood Components Number of competencies: (03)					**Number of procedures that require certification: (NIL)**		
SU3.1	Describe the indications and appropriate use of blood and blood products and complications of blood transfusion.	K	KH	Y	Lecture, Small group discussion	Written/Viva voce	
SU3.2	Observe blood transfusions.	S	SH	Y	Small group discussion, DOAP session	Skills assessment/Log book	
SU3.3	Counsel patients and family/friends for blood transfusion and blood donation.	A/C	SH	Y	DOAP session	Skills assessment	
Topic: Burns Number of competencies: (04)					**Number of procedures that require certification: (NIL)**		
SU4.1	Elicit document and present history in a case of burns and perform physical examination. Describe pathophysiology of burns.	K	KH	Y	Lecture, Small group discussion	Written/Viva voce	
SU4.2	Describe clinical features, diagnose type and extent of burns and plan appropriate treatment.	K	KH	Y	Lecture, Small group discussion	Written/Viva voce	
SU4.3	Discuss the medicolegal aspects in burn injuries.	K	KH	Y	Lecture, Small group discussion	Written/Viva voce	
SU4.4	Communicate and counsel patients and families on the outcome and rehabilitation demonstrating empathy and care.	A/C	SH	Y	Small group discussion, Role play, Skills assessment	Viva voce	
Topic: Wound Healing and Wound Care Number of competencies: (04)					**Number of procedures that require certification: (NIL)**		
SU5.1	Describe normal wound healing and factors affecting healing.	K	KH	Y	Lecture, Small group discussion	Written/Viva voce	
SU5.2	Elicit, document and present a history in a patient presenting with wounds.	C	SH	Y	Lecture, Small group discussion	Written/Viva voce	

Number	Competency: The student should be able to	Domain K/S/A/C	Level K/KH/ SH/P	Core (Y/N)	Suggested Teaching Learning method	Suggested Assessment method	Number required to certify P
SU5.3	Differentiate the various types of wounds, plan and observe management of wounds.	K	KH	Y	Lecture, Small group discussion	Written/Viva voce	
SU5.4	Discuss medicolegal aspects of wounds.	K	KH	Y	Lecture, Small group discussion	Written/Viva voce	
Topic: Surgical Infections Number of competencies: (02)					**Number of procedures that require certification: (NIL)**		
SU6.1	Define and describe the etiology and pathogenesis of surgical Infections.	K	KH	Y	Lecture, Small group discussion	Written/Viva voce	
SU6.2	Enumerate prophylactic and therapeutic antibiotics. Plan appropriate management.	K	KH	Y	Lecture, Small group discussion	Written/Viva voce	
Topic: Surgical Audit and Research Number of competencies: (02)					**Number of procedures that require certification: (NIL)**		
SU7.1	Describe the planning and conduct of surgical audit.	K	KH	Y	Lecture, Small group discussion	Written/Viva voce	
SU7.2	Describe the principles and steps of clinical research in general surgery.	K	KH	Y	Lecture, Small group discussion	Written/Viva voce	
Topic: Ethics Number of competencies: (03)					**Number of procedures that require certification: (NIL)**		
SU8.1	Describe the principles of ethics as it pertains to general surgery.	K	KH	Y	Lecture, Small group discussion	Written/Viva voce/Skill assessment	
SU8.2	Demonstrate professionalism and empathy to the patient undergoing general surgery.	A/C	SH	Y	Lecture, Small group discussion, DOAP session	Written/Viva voce/Skill assessment	
SU8.3	Discuss medicolegal issues in surgical practice.	A/C	KH	Y	Lecture, Small group discussion	Written/Viva voce/Skill assessment	
Topic: Investigation of Surgical Patient Number of competencies (03)					**Number of procedures that require certification: (NIL)**		
SU9.1	Choose appropriate biochemical, microbiological, pathological, imaging investigations and interpret the investigative data in a surgical patient.	C	KH	Y	Lecture, Small group discussion	Written/Viva voce	
SU9.2	Biological basis for early detection of cancer and multidisciplinary approach in management of cancer.	C	KH	Y	Lecture, Small group discussion	Written/Viva voce	
SU9.3	Communicate the results of surgical investigations and counsel the patient appropriately.	C	SH	Y	DOAP session	Skill assessment	
Topic: Pre, Intra and Post-operative Management Number of competencies: (04)					**Number of procedures that require certification: (NIL)**		
SU10.1	Describe the principles of perioperative management of common surgical procedures.	K	KH	Y	Lecture, Small group discussion	Written/Viva voce	
SU10.2	Describe the steps and obtain informed consent in a simulated environment.	S/A/C	SH	Y	DOAP session	Skill assessment/Log book	
SU10.3	Observe common surgical procedures and assist in minor surgical procedures; observe emergency lifesaving surgical procedures.	S	KH	Y	DOAP sessions	Log book	
SU10.4	Perform basic surgical skills such as first aid including suturing and minor surgical procedures in simulated environment.	S	P	Y	DOAP session	Skill assessment	
Topic: Anesthesia and Pain Management Number of competencies: (06)					**Number of procedures that require certification: (NIL)**		
SU11.1	Describe principles of preoperative assessment.	K	KH	Y	Lecture, Small group discussion	Written/Viva voce	
SU11.2	Enumerate the principles of general, regional, and local anesthesia.	K	KH	Y	Lecture, Small group discussion	Written/Viva voce	
SU11.3	Demonstrate maintenance of an airway in a mannequin or equivalent	S	SH	Y	DOAP session	Skill assessment	

Number	Competency: The student should be able to	Domain K/S/A/C	Level K/KH/ SH/P	Core (Y/N)	Suggested Teaching Learning method	Suggested Assessment method	Number required to certify P
SU11.4	Enumerate the indications and principles of day care general surgery	K	KH	Y	Lecture, Small group discussion	Written/Viva voce	
SU11.5	Describe principles of providing post-operative pain relief and management of chronic pain.	K	KH	Y	Lecture, Small group discussion	Written/Viva voce	
SU11.6	Describe principles of safe general surgery	K	KH	Y	Lecture, Small group discussion	Written/Viva voce	
Topic: Nutrition and Fluid Therapy			**Number of competencies: (03)**			**Number of procedures that require certification: (NIL)**	
SU12.1	Enumerate the causes and consequences of malnutrition in the surgical patient.	K	KH	Y	Lecture, Small group discussion, Bedside clinic	Written/Viva voce	
SU12.2	Describe and discuss the methods of estimation and replacement of the fluid and electrolyte requirements in the surgical patient.	K	KH	Y	Lecture, Small group discussion, Bedside clinic	Written/Viva voce	
SU12.3	Discuss the nutritional requirements of surgical patients, the methods of providing nutritional support and their complications.	K	KH	Y	Lecture, Small group discussion, Bedside clinic	Written/Viva voce	
Topic: Transplantation			**Number of competencies: (04)**			**Number of procedures that require certification: (NIL)**	
SU13.1	Describe the immunological basis of organ transplantation.	K	KH	Y	Lecture, Small group discussion	Written/Viva voce	
SU13.2	Discuss the principles of immunosuppressive therapy. Enumerate indications, describe surgical principles, management of organ transplantation.	K	KH	Y	Lecture, Small group discussion	Written/Viva voce	
SU13.3	Discuss the legal and ethical issues concerning organ donation.	K	KH	Y	Lecture, Small group discussion	Written/Viva voce	
SU13.4	Counsel patients and relatives on organ donation in a simulated environment.	S	SH	Y	DOAP session	Skill assessment	
Topic: Basic Surgical Skills			**Number of competencies: (04)**			**Number of procedures that require certification: (NIL)**	
SU14.1	Describe aseptic techniques, sterilization and disinfection.	K	KH	Y	Lecture, Small group discussion	Written/Viva voce	
SU14.2	Describe surgical approaches, incisions and the use of appropriate instruments in surgery in general.	K	KH	Y	Lecture, Small group discussion	Written/Viva voce	
SU14.3	Describe the materials and methods used for surgical wound closure and anastomosis (sutures, knots and needles).	K	KH	Y	Lecture, Small group discussion	Written/Viva voce	
SU14.4	Demonstrate the techniques of asepsis and suturing in a simulated environment.	S	SH	Y	DOAP session	Skill assessment/Log book	
Topic: Biohazard Disposal			**Number of competencies: (01)**			**Number of procedures that require certification: (NIL)**	
SU15.1	Describe classification of hospital waste and appropriate methods of disposal.	K	KH	Y	Lecture, Small group discussion	Written/Viva voce	
Topic: Minimally Invasive General Surgery			**Number of competencies: (01)**			**Number of procedures that require certification: (NIL)**	
SU16.1	Minimally invasive General Surgery: Describe indications, advantages and disadvantages of minimally invasive general surgery.	K	K	Y	Lecture, Demonstration, Bedside clinic, Discussion	Theory/ Practical/Orals/ Written/Viva voce	
Topic: Trauma			**Number of competencies: (10)**			**Number of procedures that require certification: (NIL)**	
SU17.1	Describe the principles of first aid.	S	KH	Y	Lecture, Small group discussion	Written/Viva voce	
SU17.2	Demonstrate the steps in basic life support. Transport of injured patient in a simulated environment.	S	SH	Y	DOAP session	Skill assessment	
SU17.3	Describe the principles in management of mass casualties.	K	KH	Y	Lecture, Small group discussion	Written/Viva voce	

Number	Competency: The student should be able to	Domain K/S/A/C	Level K/KH/ SH/P	Core (Y/N)	Suggested Teaching Learning method	Suggested Assessment method	Number required to certify P
SU17.4	Describe pathophysiology, mechanism of head injuries.	K	KH	Y	Lecture, Small group discussion	Written/Viva voce	
SU17.5	Describe clinical features for neurological assessment and GCS in head injuries.	K	KH	Y	Lecture, Small group discussion	Written/Viva voce	
SU17.6	Chose appropriate investigations and discuss the principles of management of head injuries.	K	KH	Y	Lecture, Small group discussion	Written/Viva voce	
SU17.7	Describe the clinical features of soft tissue injuries. Chose appropriate investigations and discuss the principles of management.	K	KH	Y	Lecture, Small group discussion	Written/Viva voce	
SU17.8	Describe the pathophysiology of chest injuries.	K	KH	Y	Lecture, Small group discussion	Written/Viva voce	
SU17.9	Describe the clinical features and principles of management of chest injuries.	K	KH	Y	Lecture, Small group discussion	Written/Viva voce	
SU17.10	Demonstrate airway maintenance. Recognize and manage tension pneumothorax, hemothorax and flail chest in simulated environment.	S	SH	Y	DOAP session	Skill assessment/Log book	

Topic: Skin and Subcutaneous Tissue   Number of competencies: (03)   Number of procedures that require certification: (NIL)

Number	Competency: The student should be able to	Domain K/S/A/C	Level K/KH/ SH/P	Core (Y/N)	Suggested Teaching Learning method	Suggested Assessment method	Number required to certify P
SU18.1	Describe the pathogenesis, clinical features and management of various cutaneous and subcutaneous infections.	K	KH	Y	Lecture, Small group discussion	Written/Viva voce	
SU18.2	Classify skin tumors. Differentiate different skin tumors and discuss their management.	K	KH	Y	Lecture, Small group discussion	Written/Viva voce/Skill assessment	
SU18.3	Describe and demonstrate the clinical examination of surgical patient including swelling and order relevant investigation for diagnosis. Describe and discuss appropriate treatment plan.	S	SH	Y	Bedside clinic, Small group discussion, DOAP session	Skill assessment	

Topic: Developmental Anomalies of Face, Mouth and Jaws   Number of competencies: (02)   Number of procedures that require certification: (NIL)

Number	Competency: The student should be able to	Domain K/S/A/C	Level K/KH/ SH/P	Core (Y/N)	Suggested Teaching Learning method	Suggested Assessment method	Number required to certify P
SU19.1	Describe the etiology and classification of cleft lip and palate.	K	KH	Y	Lecture, Small group Discussion	Written/Viva voce	
SU19.2	Describe the principles of reconstruction of cleft lip and palate.	K	KH	Y	Lecture, Small group Discussion	Written/Viva voce	

Topic: Oropharyngeal Cancer   Number of competencies: (02)   Number of procedures that require certification: (NIL)

Number	Competency: The student should be able to	Domain K/S/A/C	Level K/KH/ SH/P	Core (Y/N)	Suggested Teaching Learning method	Suggested Assessment method	Number required to certify P
SU20.1	Describe etiopathogenesis of oral cancer symptoms and signs of oropharyngeal cancer.	K	KH	Y	Lecture, Small group discussion	Written/Viva voce	
SU20.2	Enumerate the appropriate investigations and discuss the principles of treatment.	K	K	Y	Lecture, Small group discussion	Written/Viva voce	

Topic: Disorders of Salivary Glands   Number of competencies: (02)   Number of procedures that require certification: (NIL)

Number	Competency: The student should be able to	Domain K/S/A/C	Level K/KH/ SH/P	Core (Y/N)	Suggested Teaching Learning method	Suggested Assessment method	Number required to certify P
SU21.1	Describe surgical anatomy of the salivary glands, pathology, and clinical presentation of disorders of salivary glands.	K	KH	Y	Lecture, Small group discussion	Written/Viva voce	
SU21.2	Enumerate the appropriate investigations and describe the principles of treatment of disorders of salivary glands.	K	KH	Y	Lecture, Small group discussion	Written/Viva voce	

Topic: Endocrine general surgery: Thyroid and Parathyroid glands   Number of competencies: (06)   Number of procedures that require certification: (NIL)

Number	Competency: The student should be able to	Domain K/S/A/C	Level K/KH/ SH/P	Core (Y/N)	Suggested Teaching Learning method	Suggested Assessment method	Number required to certify P
SU22.1	Describe the applied anatomy and physiology of thyroid.	K	KH	Y	Lecture, Small group discussion	Written/Viva voce	
SU22.2	Describe the etiopathogenesis of thyroidal swellings.	K	KH	Y	Lecture, Small group discussion	Written/Viva voce	
SU22.3	Demonstrate and document the correct clinical examination of thyroid swellings and discuss the differential diagnosis and their management.	S	SH	Y	Bedside clinic	Skill assessment	
SU22.4	Describe the clinical features, classification and principles of management of thyroid cancer.	K	KH	Y	Lecture, Small group discussion	Written/Viva voce	

Number	Competency: The student should be able to	Domain K/S/A/C	Level K/KH/ SH/P	Core (Y/N)	Suggested Teaching Learning method	Suggested Assessment method	Number required to certify P
SU22.5	Describe the applied anatomy of parathyroid.	K	KH	Y	Lecture, Small group discussion	Written/Viva voce	
SU22.6	Describe and discuss the clinical features of hypo- and hyperparathyroidism and the principles of their management.	K	KH	Y	Lecture, Small group discussion	Written/Viva voce	
Topic: Adrenal Gland			**Number of competencies: (03)**			**Number of procedures that require certification: (NIL)**	
SU23.1	Describe the applied anatomy of adrenal gland.	K	KH	Y	Lecture, Small group discussion	Written/Viva voce	
SU23.2	Describe the etiology, clinical features and principles of management of disorders of adrenal gland.	K	KH	Y	Lecture, Small group discussion	Written/Viva voce	
SU23.3	Describe the clinical features, principles of investigation and management of adrenal tumors.	K	KH	Y	Lecture, Small group discussion, Demonstration	Written/Viva voce	
Topic: Pancreas			**Number of competencies: (03)**			**Number of procedures that require certification: (NIL)**	
SU24.1	Describe the clinical features, principles of investigation, prognosis and management of pancreatitis.	K	KH	Y	Lecture, Small group discussion	Written/Viva voce	
SU24.2	Describe the clinical features, principles of investigation, prognosis and management of pancreatic endocrine tumors.	K	KH	Y	Lecture, Small group discussion, Demonstration	Written/Viva voce	
SU24.3	Describe the principles of investigation and management of pancreatic disorders including pancreatitis and endocrine tumors.	K	KH	Y	Lecture, Small group discussion, Demonstration	Written/Viva voce/Skill assessment	
Topic: Breast			**Number of competencies: (05)**			**Number of procedures that require certification: (NIL)**	
SU25.1	Describe applied anatomy and appropriate investigations for breast disease.	K	KH	Y	Lecture, Small group discussion	Written/Viva voce/Skill assessment	
SU25.2	Describe the etiopathogenesis, clinical features and principles of management of benign breast disease including infections of the breast.	K	KH	Y	Lecture, Small group discussion	Written/Viva voce/Skill assessment	
SU25.3	Describe the etiopathogenesis, clinical features, investigations and principles of treatment of benign and malignant tumors of breast.	K	KH	Y	Lecture, Small group discussion, Demonstration	Written/Viva voce/Skill assessment	
SU25.4	Counsel the patient and obtain informed consent for treatment of malignant conditions of the breast.	A/C	SH	Y	DOAP session	Skill assessment	
SU25.5	Demonstrate the correct technique to palpate the breast for breast swelling in a mannequin or equivalent.	S	SH	Y	DOAP session	Skill assessment	
Topic: Cardiothoracic general surgery: Chest-heart and lungs			**Number of competencies: (04)**			**Number of procedures that require certification: (NIL)**	
SU26.1	Outline the role of surgery in the management of coronary heart disease, valvular heart diseases and congenital heart diseases.	K	K	Y	Lecture, Small group discussion	Written/Viva voce	
SU26.3	Describe the clinical features of mediastinal diseases and the principles of management.	K	K	Y	Lecture, Small group discussion	Written/Viva voce	
SU26.4	Describe the etiology, pathogenesis, clinical features of tumors of lung and the principles of management.	K	K	Y	Lecture, Small group discussion	Written/Viva voce	
Topic: Vascular Diseases			**Number of competencies: (08)**			**Number of procedures that require certification: (NIL)**	
SU27.1	Describe the etiopathogenesis, clinical features, investigations and principles of treatment of occlusive arterial disease.	K	KH	Y	Lecture, Small group discussion	Written/Viva voce/Skill assessment	
SU27.2	Demonstrate the correct examination of the vascular system and enumerate and describe the investigation of vascular disease.	S	SH	Y	DOAP session	Skill assessment	

Number	Competency: The student should be able to	Domain K/S/A/C	Level K/KH/ SH/P	Core (Y/N)	Suggested Teaching Learning method	Suggested Assessment method	Number required to certify P
SU27.3	Describe clinical features, investigations and principles of management of vasospastic disorders.	K	KH	Y	Lecture, Small group discussion	Written/Viva voce	
SU27.4	Describe the types of gangrene and principles of amputation.	K	KH	Y	Lecture, Small group discussion	Written/Viva voce/Skill assessment	
SU27.5	Describe the applied anatomy of venous system of lower limb.	K	K	Y	Lecture, Small group discussion	Written/Viva voce	
SU27.6	Describe pathophysiology, clinical features, investigations and principles of management of DVT and varicose veins.	K	KH	Y	Lecture, Small group discussion, Demonstration	Written/Viva voce/Skill assessment	
SU27.7	Describe pathophysiology, clinical features, investigations and principles of management of lymph edema, lymphangitis and lymphomas.	K	KH	Y	Lecture, Small group discussion	Written/Viva voce/Skill assessment	
SU27.8	Demonstrate the correct examination of the lymphatic system.	S	SH	Y	DOAP session, Bedside clinic	Skill assessment	

Topic: Abdomen   **Number of competencies: (18)**   **Number of procedures that require certification: (NIL)**

Number	Competency: The student should be able to	Domain K/S/A/C	Level K/KH/ SH/P	Core (Y/N)	Suggested Teaching Learning method	Suggested Assessment method	Number required to certify P
SU28.1	Describe pathophysiology, clinical features, investigations and principles of management of hernias.	K	KH	Y	Lecture, Small group discussion	Written/Viva voce/Skill assessment	
SU28.2	Demonstrate the correct technique to examine the patient with hernia and identify different types of hernias.	S	SH	Y	DOAP session, Bedside clinic	Skill assessment	
SU28.3	Describe causes, clinical features, complications and principles of management of peritonitis.	K	K	Y	Lecture, Small group discussion, Bedside clinic	Written/Viva voce	
SU28.4	Describe pathophysiology, clinical features, investigations and principles of management of intra-abdominal abscess, mesenteric cyst, and retroperitoneal tumors.	K	K	Y	Lecture, Small group discussion, Demonstration	Written/Viva voce	
SU28.5	Describe the applied anatomy and physiology of esophagus.	K	K	Y	Lecture, Small group discussion, Demonstration	Written/Viva voce	
SU28.6	Describe the clinical features, investigations and principles of management of benign and malignant disorders of esophagus.	K	K	Y	Lecture, Small group discussion, Demonstration	Written/Viva voce	
SU28.7	Describe the applied anatomy and physiology of stomach.	K	KH	Y	Lecture, Small group discussion	Written/Viva voce	
SU28.8	Describe and discuss the etiology, clinical features, investigations and principles of management of congenital hypertrophic pyloric stenosis, peptic ulcer disease, carcinoma stomach.	K	KH	Y	Lecture, Small group discussion	Written/Viva voce/Skill assessment	
SU28.9	Demonstrate the correct technique of examination of a patient with disorders of the stomach.	S	SH	Y	DOAP session, Bedside clinic	Skill assessment	
SU28.10	Describe the applied anatomy of liver. Describe the clinical features, investigations and principles of management of liver abscess, hydatid disease, injuries and tumors of the liver.	K	KH	Y	Lecture, Small group discussion, Demonstration	Written/Viva voce	
SU28.11	Describe the applied anatomy of spleen. Describe the clinical features, investigations and principles of management of splenic injuries. Describe the post-splenectomy sepsis—prophylaxis.	K	KH	Y	Lecture, Small group discussion, Demonstration	Written/Viva voce	
SU28.12	Describe the applied anatomy of biliary system. Describe the clinical features, investigations and principles of management of diseases of biliary system.	K	KH	Y	Lecture, Small group discussion, Demonstration	Written/Viva voce	

Number	Competency: The student should be able to	Domain K/S/A/C	Level K/KH/ SH/P	Core (Y/N)	Suggested Teaching Learning method	Suggested Assessment method	Number required to certify P
SU28.13	Describe the applied anatomy of small and large intestine.	K	KH	Y	Lecture, Small group discussion, Demonstration	Written/Viva voce	
SU28.14	Describe the clinical features, investigations and principles of management of disorders of small and large intestine including neonatal obstruction and short gut syndrome.	K	KH	Y	Lecture, Small group discussion, Demonstration	Written/Viva voce	
SU28.15	Describe the clinical features, investigations and principles of management of diseases of appendix including appendicitis and its complications.	K	KH	Y	Lecture, Small group discussion, Demonstration	Written/Viva voce/Skill assessment	
SU28.16	Describe applied anatomy including congenital anomalies of the rectum and anal canal.	K	KH	Y	Lecture, Small group discussion, Demonstration	Written/Viva voce/Skill assessment	
SU28.17	Describe the clinical features, investigations and principles of management of common anorectal diseases.	K	KH	Y	Lecture, Small group discussion, Demonstration	Written/Viva voce/Skill assessment	
SU28.18	Describe and demonstrate clinical examination of abdomen. Order relevant investigations. Describe and discuss appropriate treatment plan.	S	SH	Y	Bedside clinic, DOAP session, Small group discussion	Skill assessment	
Topic: Urinary System			**Number of competencies: (11)**			**Number of procedures that require certification: (NIL)**	
SU29.1	Describe the causes, investigations and principles of management of hematuria.	K	KH	Y	Lecture, Small group discussion	Written/Viva voce	
SU29.2	Describe the clinical features, investigations and principles of management of congenital anomalies of genitourinary system.	K	KH	Y	Lecture, Small group discussion	Written/Viva voce	
SU29.3	Describe the clinical features, investigations and principles of management of urinary tract infections.	K	KH	Y	Lecture, Small group discussion	Written/Viva voce	
SU29.4	Describe the clinical features, investigations and principles of management of hydronephrosis.	K	KH	Y	Lecture, Small group discussion	Written/Viva voce	
SU29.5	Describe the clinical features, investigations and principles of management of renal calculi.	K	KH	Y	Lecture, Small group discussion	Written/Viva voce	
SU29.6	Describe the clinical features, investigations and principles of management of renal tumors.	K	KH	Y	Lecture, Small group discussion	Written/Viva voce	
SU29.7	Describe the principles of management of acute and chronic retention of urine.	K	KH	Y	Lecture, Small group discussion	Written/Viva voce	
SU29.8	Describe the clinical features, investigations and principles of management of bladder cancer.	K	KH	Y	Lecture, Small group discussion	Written/Viva voce	
SU29.9	Describe the clinical features, investigations and principles of management of disorders of prostate.	K	KH	Y	Lecture, Small group discussion	Written/Viva voce/Skill assessment	
SU29.10	Demonstrate a digital rectal examination of the prostate in a mannequin or equivalent.	S	SH	Y	DOAP session	Skill assessment	
SU29.11	Describe clinical features, investigations and management of urethral strictures.	K	KH	Y	Lecture, Small group discussion, Demonstration	Written/Viva voce/Skill assessment	
Topic: Penis, Testis and Scrotum			**Number of competencies: (06)**			**Number of procedures that require certification: (NIL)**	
SU30.1	Describe the clinical features, investigations and principles of management of phimosis, paraphimosis and carcinoma penis.	K	KH	Y	Lecture, Small group discussion, Demonstration	Written/Viva voce/Skill assessment	
SU30.2	Describe the applied anatomy, clinical features, investigations and principles of management of undescended testis.	K	KH	Y	Lecture, Small group discussion, Demonstration	Written/Viva voce/Skill assessment	
SU30.3	Describe the applied anatomy, clinical features, investigations and principles of management of epididymo-orchitis.	K	KH	Y	Lecture, Small group discussion, Demonstration	Written/Viva voce/Skill assessment	

Number	Competency: The student should be able to	Domain K/S/A/C	Level K/KH/ SH/P	Core (Y/N)	Suggested Teaching Learning method	Suggested Assessment method	Number required to certify P
SU30.4	Describe the applied anatomy, clinical features, investigations and principles of management of varicocele.	K	KH	Y	Lecture, Small group discussion, Demonstration	Written/Viva voce/Skill assessment	
SU30.5	Describe the applied anatomy, clinical features, investigations and principles of management of hydrocele.	K	KH	Y	Lecture, Small group discussion, Demonstration	Written/Viva voce/Skill assessment	
SU30.6	Describe classification, clinical features, investigations and principles of management of tumors of testis.	K	KH	Y	Lecture, Small group discussion, Demonstration	Written/Viva voce/Skill assessment	
	Column C: K-Knowledge, S-Skill, A-Attitude/professionalism, C-Communication. **Column D: K-Knows, KH-Knows How, SH-Shows how, P-Performs independently,** **Column F: DOAP session-Demonstrate, Observe, Assess, Perform.** **Column H: If entry is P: indicate how many procedures must be done independently for certification/graduation.**						

ORTHOPEDICS

Number	Competency: The student should be able to	Domain K/S/A/C	Level K/KH/ SH/P	Core (Y/N)	Suggested Teaching Learning method	Suggested Assessment method	Number required to certify P
Topic: Skeletal Trauma, Poly trauma		**Number of competencies : (06)**			**Number of procedures that require certification: (NIL)**		
OR1.1	Describe and discuss the Principles of pre-hospital care and Casualty management of a trauma victim including principles of triage	K/S/A/C	K/KH	Y	Lecture with video, Small group discussion	Written/Viva voce/ OSCE/Simulation	
OR1.2	Describe and discuss the etiopathogenesis, clinical features, investigations, and principles of management of shock	K/S	K/KH	Y	Lecture	Written/Viva voce/ OSCE/Simulation	
OR1.3	Describe and discuss the etiopathogenesis, clinical features, investigations, and principles of management of soft tissue injuries	K	KH/ SH	Y	Lecture, Small group discussion	Written/OSCE	
OR1.4	Describe and discuss the Principles of management of soft tissue injuries	K	K/KH	Y	Lecture, Small group discussion	Written/ Assessment/Viva voce	
OR1.5	Describe and discuss the etiopathogenesis, clinical features, investigations, and principles of management of dislocation of major joints, shoulder, knee, hip	K	K/KH	Y	Lecture, Small group discussion, Bed side clinic	Written/Viva voce/ OSCE/Simulation	
OR1.6	Participate as a member in the team for closed reduction of shoulder dislocation/hip dislocation/ knee dislocation	K/S/A/C	SH	Y	Simulation, DOAP session	OSCE/Simulation	
Topic: Fractures		**Number of competencies : (16)**			**Number of procedures that require certification: (NIL)**		
OR2.1	Describe and discuss the mechanism of Injury, clinical features, investigations and plan management of fracture of clavicle	K/S	KH/ SH	Y	Lecture, Small group discussion, Bed side clinic	Written/Viva voce/ OSCE	
OR2.2	Describe and discuss the mechanism of Injury, clinical features, investigations and plan management of fractures of proximal humerus	K	K/KH/ SH	Y	Lecture, Small group discussion, Bed side clinic	Written/Viva voce/ OSCE	
OR2.3	Select, prescribe and communicate appropriate medications for relief of joint pain	K	KH/ SH	Y	Lecture, Small group discussion, Bed side clinic	Written/Viva voce/ OSCE	
OR2.4	Describe and discuss the mechanism of injury, clinical features, investigations and principles of management of fracture of shaft of humerus and intercondylar fracture humerus with emphasis on neurovascular deficit	K/S	K/KH	Y	Lecture, Small group discussion, Bed side clinic	Written/Viva voce/ OSCE	
OR2.5	Describe and discuss the etiopathogenesis, clinical features, mechanism of injury, investigation and principles of management of fractures of both bones forearm and Galeazzi and Monteggia injury	K	K/KH	Y	Lecture, Small group discussion, Bedside clinic	Written/Viva voce/ OSCE	

Number	Competency: The student should be able to	Domain K/S/A/C	Level K/KH/ SH/P	Core (Y/N)	Suggested Teaching Learning method	Suggested Assessment method	Number required to certify P
OR2.6	Describe and discuss the etiopathogenesis, mechanism of injury, clinical features, investigations and principles of management of fractures of distal radius	K	KH	Y	Lecture, Small group discussion, Bedside clinic	Written/Viva voce/ OSCE	
OR2.7	Describe and discuss the etiopathogenesis, mechanism of injury, clinical features, investigations and principles of management of pelvic injuries with emphasis on hemodynamic instability	K	K/KH/ SH	Y	Lecture, Small group discussion, Bedside clinic	Written/Viva voce/ OSCE	
OR2.8	Describe and discuss the etiopathogenesis, mechanism of injury, clinical features, investigations and principles of management of spine injuries with emphasis on mobilization of the patient	K	K/KH	Y	Lecture, Small group discussion, Bedside clinic	Written/Viva voce/ OSCE	
OR2.9	Describe and discuss the mechanism of injury, Clinical features, investigations and principle of management of acetabular fracture	K	K/KH	Y	Lecture, Small group discussion, Bedside clinic	Written/Viva voce/ OSCE	
OR2.10	Describe and discuss the etiopathogenesis, mechanism of injury, clinical features, investigations and principles of management of fractures of proximal femur	K/S/A/C	KH	Y	Lecture, Small group discussion, Bedside clinic	Written/Viva voce/ OSCE	
OR2.11	Describe and discuss the etiopathogenesis, mechanism of injury, clinical features, investigations and principles of management of: a. Fracture patella b. Fracture distal femur c. Fracture proximal tibia with special focus on neurovascular injury and compartment syndrome	K	K/KH	Y	Lecture, Small group discussion, Bedside clinic	Written/Viva voce/ OSCE	
OR2.12	Describe and discuss the etiopathogenesis, clinical features, investigations and principles of management of Fracture shaft of femur in all age groups and the recognition and management of fat embolism as a complication	K	K/KH	Y	Lecture, Small group discussion, Bedside clinic	Written/Viva voce/ OSCE	
OR2.13	Describe and discuss the etiopathogenesis, clinical features, Investigation and principles of management of: a. Fracture both bones leg b. Calcaneus c. Small bones of foot	K	K/KH	Y	Lecture, Small group discussion, Bedside clinic	Written/Viva voce/ OSCE	
OR2.14	Describe and discuss the etiopathogenesis, clinical features, Investigation and principles of management of ankle fractures	K/S/C	K/KH	Y	Lecture, Small group discussion, Bedside clinic	Written/Viva voce/ OSCE	
OR2.15	Plan and interpret the investigations to diagnose complications of fractures like malunion, non-union, infection, compartmental syndrome	K/S	SH	Y	Lecture, Small group discussion, Bedside clinic	Written/Viva voce/ OSCE	
OR2.16	Describe and discuss the mechanism of injury, clinical features, investigations and principles of management of open fractures with focus on secondary infection prevention and management	K	K/KH	Y	Lecture, Small group discussion, Bedside clinic	Written/Viva voce/ OSCE	
Topic: Musculoskeletal Infection		**Number of competencies : (03)**				**Number of procedures that require certification: (NIL)**	
OR3.1	Describe and discuss the etiopathogenesis, clinical features, investigations and principles of management of Bone and Joint infections: a. Acute Osteomyelitis b. Subacute osteomyelitis c. Acute Suppurative arthritis d. Septic arthritis and HIV infection e. Spirochaetal infection f. Skeletal Tuberculosis	K/S	K/KH/ SH	Y	Lecture, Small group discussion, Video assisted lecture	Written/Viva voce/ OSCE	

Number	Competency: The student should be able to	Domain K/S/A/C	Level K/KH/ SH/P	Core (Y/N)	Suggested Teaching Learning method	Suggested Assessment method	Number required to certify P
OR3.2	Participate as a member in team for aspiration of joints under supervision	K/S/A/C	SH	Y	Small group Discussion. DOAP session	Viva voce/OSCE/ Skills assessment	
OR3.3	Participate as a member in team for procedures like drainage of abscess, sequestrectomy/ saucerization and arthrotomy	K/S/A/C	SH	Y	DOAP session, Video demonstration	Viva voce/OSCE/ Skills assessment	
Topic: Skeletal Tuberculosis Number of competencies : (01) Number of procedures that require certification: (NIL)							
OR4.1	Describe and discuss the clinical features, Investigation and principles of management of Tuberculosis affecting major joints (Hip, Knee) including cold abscess and caries spine	K	K/KH	Y	Lecture, Small group discussion, Case discussion	Written/Viva voce/ OSCE	
Topic: Rheumatoid Arthritis and associated inflammatory disorders Number of competencies : (01) Number of procedures that require certification: (NIL)							
OR5.1	Describe and discuss the etiopathogenesis, clinical features, investigations and principles of management of various inflammatory disorder of joints	K	K/KH	Y	Lecture, Small group discussion, Bedside clinic	Written/Viva voce/ OSCE	
Topic: Degenerative disorders Number of competencies : (01) Number of procedures that require certification: (NIL)							
OR6.1	Describe and discuss the clinical features, investigations and principles of management of degenerative condition of spine (Cervical Spondylosis, Lumbar Spondylosis, PID)	K	K/KH	Y	Lecture, Small group discussion, Case discussion	Written/Viva voce/ OSCE	
Topic: Metabolic bone disorders Number of competencies : (01) Number of procedures that require certification: (NIL)							
OR7.1	Describe and discuss the etiopathogenesis, clinical features, investigation and principles of management of metabolic bone disorders in particular osteoporosis, osteomalacia, rickets, Paget's disease	K	K/KH	Y	Lecture, Small group discussion, Case discussion	Written/Viva voce/ OSCE	
Topic: Poliomyelitis Number of competencies : (01) Number of procedures that require certification: (NIL)							
OR8.1	Describe and discuss the etiopathogenesis, clinical features, assessment and principles of management a patient with Post-Polio Residual Paralysis	K	K/KH	Y	Lecture, Small group discussion, Case discussion	Written/Viva voce/ OSCE	
Topic: Cerebral Palsy Number of competencies : (01) Number of procedures that require certification: (NIL)							
OR9.1	Describe and discuss the etiopathogenesis, clinical features, assessment and principles of management of cerebral palsy patient	K	K/KH	Y	Lecture, Small group discussion	Written/Viva voce/ OSCE	
Topic: Bone Tumors Number of competencies : (01) Number of procedures that require certification: (NIL)							
OR10.1	Describe and discuss the etiopathogenesis, clinical features, investigations and principles of management of benign and malignant bone tumors and pathological fractures	K	K/KH	Y	Lecture, Small group discussion, Video assisted interactive lecture	Written/Viva voce/ OSCE	
Topic: Peripheral nerve injuries Number of competencies : (01) Number of procedures that require certification: (NIL)							
OR11.1	Describe and discuss the etiopathogenesis, clinical features, investigations and principles of management of peripheral nerve injuries in diseases like foot drop, wrist drop, claw hand, palsies of radial, ulnar, median, lateral popliteal and sciatic nerves	K	K/H	Y	Lecture, Small group discussion, case discussion	Written/Viva voce/ OSCE	
Topic: Congenital lesions Number of competencies : (01) Number of procedures that require certification: (NIL)							
OR12.1	Describe and discuss the clinical features, investigations and principles of management of Congenital and acquired malformations and deformities of: a. Limbs and spine—Scoliosis and spinal bifida b. Congenital dislocation of hip, torticollis, c. Congenital talipes equinovarus	K	KH	Y	Lecture, Small group discussion	Written/Viva voce/ OSCE	

Number	Competency: The student should be able to	Domain K/S/A/C	Level K/KH/ SH/P	Core (Y/N)	Suggested Teaching Learning method	Suggested Assessment method	Number required to certify P
Topic: Procedural Skills		**Number of competencies : (02)**			**Number of procedures that require certification: (NIL)**		
OR13.1	Participate in a team for procedures in patients and demonstrating the ability to perform on mannequins/simulated patients in the following: a. Above elbow plaster b. Below knee plaster c. Above knee plaster d. Thomas splint e. Splinting for long bone fractures f. Strapping for shoulder and clavicle trauma	S/A	KH/ SH	Y	Case discussion, Video assisted Lecture, Small group discussion, Teaching, Skill lab sessions	OSCE with Simulation based assessment	
OR13.2	Participate as a member in team for Resuscitation of Polytrauma victim by doing all of the following: a. IV access central-peripheral b. Bladder catheterization c. Endotracheal intubation d. Splintage	S/A	KH/ SH	Y	Case discussion, Video assisted Lecture, Small group discussion, Teaching, Skill lab sessions	OSCE with Simulation based assessment	
Topic: Counselling Skills		**Number of competencies : (03)**			**Number of procedures that require certification: (NIL)**		
OR14.1	Demonstrate the ability to counsel patients regarding prognosis in patients with various orthopedic illnesses like a. Fractures with disabilities b. Fractures that require prolonged bed stay c. Bone tumors d. Congenital disabilities	K/S/A/C	KH/ SH	Y	Case discussion, Video assisted lecture, Small group discussion, Teaching, Skills lab sessions	OSCE with Simulation based assessment	
OR14.2	Demonstrate the ability to counsel patients to obtain consent for various orthopedic procedures like limp amputation, permanent fixations etc..	K/S/A/C	KH/ SH	Y	Case discussion, Video assisted Lecture, Small group discussion, Teaching, Skills lab sessions	OSCE with Simulation based assessment	
OR14.3	Demonstrate the ability to convince the patient for referral to a higher center in various orthopedic illnesses, based on the detection of warning signals and need for sophisticated management	K/S/A/C	KH/ SH	Y	Case discussion, Video assisted Lecture, Small group discussion, Teaching, Skills lab sessions	OSCE with Simulation based assessment	
	Column C: K-Knowledge, S-Skill, A-Attitude/professionalism, C-Communication. **Column D: K-Knows, KH-Knows How, SH-Shows how, P-Performs independently,** **Column F: DOAP session-Demonstrate, Observe, Assess, Perform.** **Column H: If entry is P: indicate how many procedures must be done independently for certification/graduation.**						

ANESTHESIOLOGY

Number	Competency: The student should be able to	Domain K/S/A/C	Level K/KH/ SH/P	Core (Y/N)	Suggested Teaching Learning method	Suggested Assessment method	Number required to certify P
Topic: Anesthesiology as a specialty		**Number of competencies: (04)**			**Number of procedures that require certification: (NIL)**		
AS1.1	Describe the evolution of Anesthesiology as a modern specialty	K	K	N	Lecture	Written/Viva voce	
AS1.2	Describe the roles of Anesthesiologist in the medical profession (including as a perioperative physician, in the intensive care and high dependency units, in the management of acute and chronic pain, including labor analgesia, in the resuscitation of acutely ill)	K	K	N	Lecture	Written/Viva voce	
AS1.3	Enumerate and describe the principle of ethics as it relates to Anesthesiology	K	K	N	Lecture	Written/Viva voce	
AS1.4	Describe the prospects of Anesthesiology as a career	K	K	N	Lecture	Written/Viva voce	

Number	Competency: The student should be able to	Domain K/S/A/C	Level K/KH/ SH/P	Core (Y/N)	Suggested Teaching Learning method	Suggested Assessment method	Number required to certify P
Topic: Cardiopulmonary resuscitation		Number of competencies: (02)			Number of procedures that require certification : (NIL)		
AS2.1	Enumerate the indications, describe the steps and demonstrate in a simulated environment, Basic Life Support in adults, children and neonates	K/S	SH	N	DOAP session	Skill assessment	
AS2.2	Enumerate the indications, describe the steps and demonstrate in a simulated environment, Advanced Life Support in adults and children	S	SH	N	DOAP session	Skill assessment	
Topic: Preoperative evaluation and medication		Number of competencies: (06)			Number of procedures that require certification : (NIL)		
AS3.1	Describe the principles of preoperative evaluation	K	KH	Y	Lecture, Small group discussion	Written/Viva voce	
AS3.2	Elicit, present and document an appropriate history including medication history in a patient undergoing surgery as it pertains to a preoperative anesthetic evaluation	S	SH	Y	DOAP session, Bedside clinic	Skill station	
AS3.3	Demonstrate and document an appropriate clinical examination in a patient undergoing general surgery	S	SH	Y	DOAP session, Bedside clinic	Skill station	
AS3.4	Choose and interpret appropriate testing for patients undergoing surgery	S	SH	Y	DOAP session, Bedside clinic	Skill station	
AS3.5	Determine the readiness for general surgery in a patient based on the preoperative evaluation	S	SH	Y	DOAP session, Bedside clinic	Skill station	
AS3.6	Choose and write a prescription for appropriate premedications for patients undergoing surgery	S	SH	Y	DOAP session, Bedside clinic	Skill station	
Topic: General Anesthesia		Number of competencies: (07)			Number of procedures that require certification : (NIL)		
AS4.1	Describe and discuss the pharmacology of drugs used in induction and maintenance of general anesthesia (including intravenous and inhalation induction agents, opiate and non-opiate analgesics, depolarizing and non-depolarizing muscle relaxants, anticholinesterases)	K	KH	Y	Lecture, Small group discussion	Written/Viva voce	
AS4.2	Describe the anatomy of the airway and its implications for general anesthesia	K	KH	Y	Lecture, Small group discussion	Written/Viva voce	
AS4.3	Observe and describe the principles and the practical aspects of induction and maintenance of anesthesia	S	KH	Y	Lecture, Small group discussion, DOAP session	Written/Viva voce	
AS4.4	Observe and describe the principles and the steps/techniques in maintenance of vital organ functions in patients undergoing surgical procedures	S	KH	Y	Lecture, Small group discussion, DOAP session	Written/Viva voce	
AS4.5	Observe and describe the principles and the steps/techniques in monitoring patients during anesthesia	S	KH	Y	Lecture, Small group discussion, DOAP session	Written/Viva voce	
AS4.6	Observe and describe the principles and the steps/techniques involved in day care anesthesia	S	KH	Y	Lecture, Small group discussion, DOAP session	Written/Viva voce	
AS4.7	Observe and describe the principles and the steps/techniques involved in anesthesia outside the operating room	S	KH	Y	Lecture, Small group discussion, DOAP session	Written/Viva voce	
Topic: Regional anesthesia		Number of competencies: (06)			Number of procedures that require certification: (NIL)		
AS5.1	Enumerate the indications for and describe the principles of regional anesthesia (including spinal, epidural and combined)	K	KH	Y	Lecture, Small group discussion	Written/Viva voce	
AS5.2	Describe the correlative anatomy of the brachial plexus, subarachnoid and epidural spaces	K	KH	Y	Lecture, Small group discussion	Written/Viva voce	
AS5.3	Observe and describe the principles and steps/techniques involved in peripheral nerve blocks	S	KH	Y	Lecture, Small group discussion, DOAP session	Written/Viva voce	

Number	Competency: The student should be able to	Domain K/S/A/C	Level K/KH/ SH/P	Core (Y/N)	Suggested Teaching Learning method	Suggested Assessment method	Number required to certify P
AS5.4	Observe and describe the pharmacology and correct use of commonly used drugs and adjuvant agents in regional anesthesia	S	KH	Y	Lecture, Small group discussion, DOAP session	Written/Viva voce	
AS5.5	Observe and describe the principles and steps/techniques involved in caudal epidural in adults and children	S	KH	Y	Lecture, Small group discussion, DOAP session	Written/Viva voce	
AS5.6	Observe and describe the principles and steps/techniques involved in common blocks used in surgery (including brachial plexus blocks)	S	KH	Y	Lecture, Small group discussion, DOAP session	Written/Viva voce	
Topic: Post-anesthesia recovery		**Number of competencies: (03)**			**Number of procedures that require certification: (NIL)**		
AS6.1	Describe the principles of monitoring and resuscitation in the recovery room	S	KH	Y	Lecture, Small group discussion, DOAP session	Written/Viva voce	
AS6.2	Observe and enumerate the contents of the crash cart and describe the equipment used in the recovery room	S	KH	Y	Lecture, Small group discussion, DOAP session	Written/Viva voce	
AS6.3	Describe the common complications encountered by patients in the recovery room, their recognition and principles of management	K	KH	Y	Lecture, Small group discussion, DOAP session	Written/Viva voce	
Topic: Intensive Care Management		**Number of competencies: (05)**			**Number of procedures that require certification: (NIL)**		
AS7.1	Visit, enumerate and describe the functions of an Intensive Care Unit	S	KH	Y	Lecture, Small group discussion, DOAP session	Written/Viva voce	
AS7.2	Enumerate and describe the criteria for admission and discharge of a patient to an ICU	S	KH	Y	Lecture, Small group discussion, DOAP session	Written/Viva voce	
AS7.3	Observe and describe the management of an unconscious patient	S	KH	Y	Lecture, Small group discussion, DOAP session	Written/Viva voce	
AS7.4	Observe and describe the basic setup process of a ventilator	S	KH	Y	Lecture, Small group discussion, DOAP session	Written/Viva voce	
AS7.5	Observe and describe the principles of monitoring in an ICU	S	KH	Y	Lecture, Small group discussion, DOAP session	Written/Viva voce	
Topic: Pain and its management		**Number of competencies: (05)**			**Number of procedures that require certification: (NIL)**		
AS8.1	Describe the anatomical correlates and physiologic principles of pain	K	KH	Y	Lecture, Small group discussion, DOAP session	Written/Viva voce	
AS8.2	Elicit and determine the level, quality and quantity of pain and its tolerance in patient or surrogate	S	KH	Y	Lecture, Small group discussion, DOAP session	Written/Viva voce	
AS8.3	Describe the pharmacology and use of drugs in the management of pain	K	KH	Y	Lecture, Small group discussion, DOAP session	Written/Viva voce	
AS8.4	Describe the principles of pain management in palliative care	K	KH	Y	Lecture, Small group discussion, DOAP session	Written/Viva voce	
AS8.5	Describe the principles of pain management in the terminally ill	K	KH	Y	Lecture, Small group discussion, DOAP session	Written/Viva voce	
Topic: Fluids		**Number of competencies: (04)**			**Number of procedures that require certification: (NIL)**		
AS9.1	Establish intravenous access in a simulated environment	S	KH	Y	Small group discussion, DOAP session	Skill assessment	
AS9.2	Establish central venous access in a simulated environment	S	KH	Y	Small group discussion, DOAP session	Skill assessment	
AS9.3	Describe the principles of fluid therapy in the preoperative period	K	KH	Y	Lecture, Small group discussion, DOAP session	Written/Viva voce	
AS9.4	Enumerate blood products and describe the use of blood products in the preoperative period	K	KH	Y	Lecture, Small group discussion, DOAP session	Written/Viva voce	
Topic: Patient safety		**Number of competencies: (04)**			**Number of procedures that require certification: (NIL)**		
AS10.1	Enumerate the hazards of incorrect patient positioning	K	KH	Y	Lecture, Small group discussion, DOAP session	Written/Viva voce	
AS10.2	Enumerate the hazards encountered in the perioperative period and steps/techniques taken to prevent them	K	KH	Y	Lecture, Small group discussion, DOAP session	Written/Viva voce	

Number	Competency: The student should be able to	Domain K/S/A/C	Level K/KH/ SH/P	Core (Y/N)	Suggested Teaching Learning method	Suggested Assessment method	Number required to certify P
AS10.3	Describe the role of communication in patient safety	K	KH	Y	Lecture, Small group discussion, DOAP session	Written/Viva voce	
AS10.4	Define and describe common medical and medication errors in anesthesia	K	KH	Y	Lecture, Small group discussion, DOAP session	Written/Viva voce	
	Column C: K-Knowledge, S-Skill, A-Attitude/professionalism, C-Communication. **Column D: K-Knows, KH-Knows How, SH-Shows how, P-Performs independently,** **Column F: DOAP session-Demonstrate, Observe, Assess, Perform.** **Column H: If entry is P: indicate how many procedures must be done independently for certification/graduation.**						

RADIODIAGNOSIS

Number	Competency: The student should be able to	Domain K/S/A/C	Level K/KH/ SH/P	Core (Y/N)	Suggested Teaching Learning method	Suggested Assessment method	Number required to certify P
Topic: Radiological investigations and Radiation safety Number of competencies: (13) Number of procedures that require certification: (NIL)							
RD1.1	Define radiation and the interaction of radiation and importance of radiation protection	K	KH	Y	Lecture, Demonstration		
RD1.2	Describe the evolution of Radiodiagnosis. Identify various radiological equipments In the current era	S	SH	Y	Lecture, Demonstration		
RD1.3	Enumerate indications for various common radiological investigations, choose the most appropriate and cost effective method and interpret findings in common conditions pertaining to disorder of ENT	K/S	SH	Y	Lecture, Demonstration		
RD1.4	Enumerate indications for various common radiological investigations, choose the most appropriate and cost effective method and interpret findings in common conditions pertaining to disorder in Obstetrics and Gynecology	K/S	SH	Y	Lecture, Demonstration		
RD1.5	Enumerate indications for various common radiological investigations, choose the most appropriate and cost effective method and interpret findings in common conditions pertaining to disorder in internal medicine	K/S	SH	Y	Lecture, Demonstration		
RD1.6	Enumerate indications for various common radiological investigations, choose the most appropriate and cost effective method and interpret findings in common conditions pertaining to disorders in surgery	K/S	SH	Y	Lecture, Demonstration		
RD1.7	Enumerate indications for various common radiological investigations, choose the most appropriate and cost effective method and interpret findings in common conditions pertaining to disorder in Pediatrics	K/S	SH	Y	Lecture, Demonstration		
RD1.8	Enumerate indications for various common radiological investigations, choose the most appropriate and cost effective method and interpret findings in common conditions pertaining to common malignancies	K/S	SH	Y	Lecture, Demonstration		
RD1.9	Describe the role of Interventional Radiology in common clinical conditions	K	KH	Y	Lecture, Demonstration		
RD1.10	Describe the role of Emergency Radiology, miscellaneous and applied aspects, interaction with clinical departments	K	KH	Y	Lecture, Demonstration		
RD1.11	Describe preparation of patient for common imaging procedures	K	KH	Y	Lecture, Demonstration		

Number	Competency: The student should be able to	Domain K/S/A/C	Level K/KH/ SH/P	Core (Y/N)	Suggested Teaching Learning method	Suggested Assessment method	Number required to certify P
RD1.12	Describe the effects of radiation in pregnancy and the methods of prevention/minimization of radiation exposure	K	KH	Y	Lecture, Demonstration		
RD1.13	Describe the components of the PC and PNDT Act and its medicolegal implications	K	KH	Y	Lecture, Small group discussion		
	Column C: K-Knowledge, S-Skill, A-Attitude/professionalism, C-Communication. **Column D: K-Knows, KH-Knows How, SH-Shows how, P-Performs independently,** **Column F: DOAP session-Demonstrate, Observe, Assess, Perform.** **Column H: If entry is P: indicate how many procedures must be done independently for certification/graduation.**						

GENERAL SURGERY

SU1: METABOLIC RESPONSE TO SURGERY

METABOLIC RESPONSE TO SURGERY						
Name of Activity	Date Completed (dd-mm-yyyy)	Attempt at activity First (F) Repeat (R) Remedial (Re)	Rating Below (B) Meets (M) Exceeds (E) Expectations	Decision of Faculty Complete (C) Repeat (R) Remedial (Re)	Initial of Faculty and Date	Feedback Received Initial of Learner

SU2: SHOCK

SHOCK						
SU2.3: Communicate and counsel patients and families about the treatment and prognosis of shock demonstrating empathy and care.						
Name of Activity	*Date Completed (dd-mm-yyyy)*	*Attempt at activity First (F) Repeat (R) Remedial (Re)*	*Rating Below (B) Meets (M) Exceeds (E) Expectations*	*Decision of Faculty Complete (C) Repeat (R) Remedial (Re)*	*Initial of Faculty and Date*	*Feedback Received Initial of Learner*

		SHOCK				
Name of Activity	Date Completed (dd-mm-yyyy)	Attempt at activity First (F) Repeat (R) Remedial (Re)	Rating Below (B) Meets (M) Exceeds (E) Expectations	Decision of Faculty Complete (C) Repeat (R) Remedial (Re)	Initial of Faculty and Date	Feedback Received Initial of Learner

SU3: BLOOD AND BLOOD COMPONENTS

BLOOD AND BLOOD COMPONENTS

SU3.2: Observe blood transfusions.

Name of Activity	Date Completed (dd-mm-yyyy)	Attempt at activity First (F) Repeat (R) Remedial (Re)	Rating Below (B) Meets (M) Exceeds (E) Expectations	Decision of Faculty Complete (C) Repeat (R) Remedial (Re)	Initial of Faculty and Date	Feedback Received Initial of Learner

BLOOD AND BLOOD COMPONENTS

SU3.3: Counsel patients and family/friends for blood transfusion and blood donation.

Name of Activity	Date Completed (dd-mm-yyyy)	Attempt at activity First (F) Repeat (R) Remedial (Re)	Rating Below (B) Meets (M) Exceeds (E) Expectations	Decision of Faculty Complete (C) Repeat (R) Remedial (Re)	Initial of Faculty and Date	Feedback Received Initial of Learner

BLOOD AND BLOOD COMPONENTS

Name of Activity	Date Completed (dd-mm-yyyy)	Attempt at activity First (F) Repeat (R) Remedial (Re)	Rating Below (B) Meets (M) Exceeds (E) Expectations	Decision of Faculty Complete (C) Repeat (R) Remedial (Re)	Initial of Faculty and Date	Feedback Received Initial of Learner

SU4: BURNS

BURNS						
SU4.1: Elicit document and present history in a case of burns and perform physical examination.						
Name of Activity	Date Completed (dd-mm-yyyy)	Attempt at activity First (F) Repeat (R) Remedial (Re)	Rating Below (B) Meets (M) Exceeds (E) Expectations	Decision of Faculty Complete (C) Repeat (R) Remedial (Re)	Initial of Faculty and Date	Feedback Received Initial of Learner

BURNS						
SU4.4: Communicate and counsel patients and families on the outcome and rehabilitation demonstrating empathy and care (should be able to communicate and counsel regarding burns, the nature of injury, severity and outcomes, the treatment plan).						
Name of Activity	Date Completed (dd-mm-yyyy)	Attempt at activity First (F) Repeat (R) Remedial (Re)	Rating Below (B) Meets (M) Exceeds (E) Expectations	Decision of Faculty Complete (C) Repeat (R) Remedial (Re)	Initial of Faculty and Date	Feedback Received Initial of Learner

BURNS

Name of Activity	Date Completed (dd-mm-yyyy)	Attempt at activity First (F) Repeat (R) Remedial (Re)	Rating Below (B) Meets (M) Exceeds (E) Expectations	Decision of Faculty Complete (C) Repeat (R) Remedial (Re)	Initial of Faculty and Date	Feedback Received Initial of Learner

SU5 : WOUND HEALING AND WOUND CARE

WOUND HEALING AND WOUND CARE						

SU5.2: Elicit, document and present a history in a patient presenting with wounds.
1. Should be able to elicit history to find out the cause and type of ulcer or wound
2. Should be able to describe the wound and subsequent plan of management

Name of Activity	Date Completed (dd-mm-yyyy)	Attempt at activity First (F) Repeat (R) Remedial (Re)	Rating Below (B) Meets (M) Exceeds (E) Expectations	Decision of Faculty Complete (C) Repeat (R) Remedial (Re)	Initial of Faculty and Date	Feedback Received Initial of Learner

WOUND HEALING AND WOUND CARE						
Name of Activity	Date Completed (dd-mm-yyyy)	Attempt at activity First (F) Repeat (R) Remedial (Re)	Rating Below (B) Meets (M) Exceeds (E) Expectations	Decision of Faculty Complete (C) Repeat (R) Remedial (Re)	Initial of Faculty and Date	Feedback Received Initial of Learner

SU6: SURGICAL INFECTIONS

			SURGICAL INFECTIONS			
Name of Activity	Date Completed (dd-mm-yyyy)	Attempt at activity First (F) Repeat (R) Remedial (Re)	Rating Below (B) Meets (M) Exceeds (E) Expectations	Decision of Faculty Complete (C) Repeat (R) Remedial (Re)	Initial of Faculty and Date	Feedback Received Initial of Learner

SU7: SURGICAL AUDIT AND RESEARCH

SURGICAL AUDIT AND RESEARCH						
Name of Activity	*Date Completed (dd-mm-yyyy)*	*Attempt at activity First (F) Repeat (R) Remedial (Re)*	*Rating Below (B) Meets (M) Exceeds (E) Expectations*	*Decision of Faculty Complete (C) Repeat (R) Remedial (Re)*	*Initial of Faculty and Date*	*Feedback Received Initial of Learner*

ETHICS

SU8.3: Discuss medicolegal issues in surgical practice.

Name of Activity	Date Completed (dd-mm-yyyy)	Attempt at activity First (F) Repeat (R) Remedial (Re)	Rating Below (B) Meets (M) Exceeds (E) Expectations	Decision of Faculty Complete (C) Repeat (R) Remedial (Re)	Initial of Faculty and Date	Feedback Received Initial of Learner

ETHICS						
Name of Activity	Date Completed (dd-mm-yyyy)	Attempt at activity First (F) Repeat (R) Remedial (Re)	Rating Below (B) Meets (M) Exceeds (E) Expectations	Decision of Faculty Complete (C) Repeat (R) Remedial (Re)	Initial of Faculty and Date	Feedback Received Initial of Learner

SU10: PRE, INTRA AND POST-OPERATIVE MANAGEMENT

PRE, INTRA AND POST-OPERATIVE MANAGEMENT

SU10.3: Observe common surgical procedures and assist in minor surgical procedures; observe emergency lifesaving surgical procedures.

Name of Activity	Date Completed (dd-mm-yyyy)	Attempt at activity First (F) Repeat (R) Remedial (Re)	Rating Below (B) Meets (M) Exceeds (E) Expectations	Decision of Faculty Complete (C) Repeat (R) Remedial (Re)	Initial of Faculty and Date	Feedback Received Initial of Learner

PRE, INTRA AND POST-OPERATIVE MANAGEMENT

SU10.4: Perform basic surgical Skills such as first aid including suturing and minor surgical procedures in simulated environment.

Name of Activity	Date Completed (dd-mm-yyyy)	Attempt at activity First (F) Repeat (R) Remedial (Re)	Rating Below (B) Meets (M) Exceeds (E) Expectations	Decision of Faculty Complete (C) Repeat (R) Remedial (Re)	Initial of Faculty and Date	Feedback Received Initial of Learner

SU12: NUTRITION AND FLUID THERAPY

NUTRITION AND FLUID THERAPY						
Name of Activity	Date Completed (dd-mm-yyyy)	Attempt at activity First (F) Repeat (R) Remedial (Re)	Rating Below (B) Meets (M) Exceeds (E) Expectations	Decision of Faculty Complete (C) Repeat (R) Remedial (Re)	Initial of Faculty and Date	Feedback Received Initial of Learner

SU13: TRANSPLANTATION

TRANSPLANTATION						
SU13.4: Counsel patients and relatives on organ donation in a simulated environment.						
Name of Activity	*Date Completed (dd-mm-yyyy)*	*Attempt at activity First (F) Repeat (R) Remedial (Re)*	*Rating Below (B) Meets (M) Exceeds (E) Expectations*	*Decision of Faculty Complete (C) Repeat (R) Remedial (Re)*	*Initial of Faculty and Date*	*Feedback Received Initial of Learner*

SU15: BIOHAZARD DISPOSAL

BIOHAZARD DISPOSAL						
Name of Activity	Date Completed (dd-mm-yyyy)	Attempt at activity First (F) Repeat (R) Remedial (Re)	Rating Below (B) Meets (M) Exceeds (E) Expectations	Decision of Faculty Complete (C) Repeat (R) Remedial (Re)	Initial of Faculty and Date	Feedback Received Initial of Learner

SU16: MINIMALLY INVASIVE GENERAL SURGERY

MINIMALLY INVASIVE GENERAL SURGERY						
Name of Activity	Date Completed (dd-mm-yyyy)	Attempt at activity First (F) Repeat (R) Remedial (Re)	Rating Below (B) Meets (M) Exceeds (E) Expectations	Decision of Faculty Complete (C) Repeat (R) Remedial (Re)	Initial of Faculty and Date	Feedback Received Initial of Learner

SU17: TRAUMA

TRAUMA						
SU17.10: Demonstrate airway maintenance. Recognize and manage tension pneumothorax, hemothorax and flail chest in simulated environment.						
Name of Activity	*Date Completed (dd-mm-yyyy)*	*Attempt at activity First (F) Repeat (R) Remedial (Re)*	*Rating Below (B) Meets (M) Exceeds (E) Expectations*	*Decision of Faculty Complete (C) Repeat (R) Remedial (Re)*	*Initial of Faculty and Date*	*Feedback Received Initial of Learner*

TRAUMA						
SU17.2: Demonstrate the steps in basic life support. Transport of injured patient in a simulated environment.						
Name of Activity	Date Completed (dd-mm-yyyy)	Attempt at activity First (F) Repeat (R) Remedial (Re)	Rating Below (B) Meets (M) Exceeds (E) Expectations	Decision of Faculty Complete (C) Repeat (R) Remedial (Re)	Initial of Faculty and Date	Feedback Received Initial of Learner

TRAUMA						
Name of Activity	Date Completed (dd-mm-yyyy)	Attempt at activity First (F) Repeat (R) Remedial (Re)	Rating Below (B) Meets (M) Exceeds (E) Expectations	Decision of Faculty Complete (C) Repeat (R) Remedial (Re)	Initial of Faculty and Date	Feedback Received Initial of Learner

SU18: SKIN AND SUBCUTANEOUS TISSUE

SKIN AND SUBCUTANEOUS TISSUE

SU18.2: Classify skin tumors. Differentiate different skin tumors and discuss their management.

Name of Activity	Date Completed (dd-mm-yyyy)	Attempt at activity First (F) Repeat (R) Remedial (Re)	Rating Below (B) Meets (M) Exceeds (E) Expectations	Decision of Faculty Complete (C) Repeat (R) Remedial (Re)	Initial of Faculty and Date	Feedback Received Initial of Learner

SKIN AND SUBCUTANEOUS TISSUE

SU18.3: Describe and demonstrate the clinical examination of surgical patient including swelling and order relevant investigation for diagnosis. Describe and discuss appropriate treatment plan.

Name of Activity	Date Completed (dd-mm-yyyy)	Attempt at activity First (F) Repeat (R) Remedial (Re)	Rating Below (B) Meets (M) Exceeds (E) Expectations	Decision of Faculty Complete (C) Repeat (R) Remedial (Re)	Initial of Faculty and Date	Feedback Received Initial of Learner

SKIN AND SUBCUTANEOUS TISSUE						
Name of Activity	Date Completed (dd-mm-yyyy)	Attempt at activity First (F) Repeat (R) Remedial (Re)	Rating Below (B) Meets (M) Exceeds (E) Expectations	Decision of Faculty Complete (C) Repeat (R) Remedial (Re)	Initial of Faculty and Date	Feedback Received Initial of Learner

SU19: DEVELOPMENTAL ANOMALIES OF FACE, MOUTH AND JAWS

DEVELOPMENTAL ANOMALIES OF FACE, MOUTH AND JAWS						
Name of Activity	Date Completed (dd-mm-yyyy)	Attempt at activity First (F) Repeat (R) Remedial (Re)	Rating Below (B) Meets (M) Exceeds (E) Expectations	Decision of Faculty Complete (C) Repeat (R) Remedial (Re)	Initial of Faculty and Date	Feedback Received Initial of Learner

SU20: OROPHARYNGEAL CANCER

	OROPHARYNGEAL CANCER					
Name of Activity	Date Completed (dd-mm-yyyy)	Attempt at activity First (F) Repeat (R) Remedial (Re)	Rating Below (B) Meets (M) Exceeds (E) Expectations	Decision of Faculty Complete (C) Repeat (R) Remedial (Re)	Initial of Faculty and Date	Feedback Received Initial of Learner

SU21: DISORDERS OF THE SALIVARY GLANDS

DISORDERS OF THE SALIVARY GLANDS						
Name of Activity	Date Completed (dd-mm-yyyy)	Attempt at activity First (F) Repeat (R) Remedial (Re)	Rating Below (B) Meets (M) Exceeds (E) Expectations	Decision of Faculty Complete (C) Repeat (R) Remedial (Re)	Initial of Faculty and Date	Feedback Received Initial of Learner

SU22: THYROID AND PARATHYROID GLANDS

THYROID AND PARATHYROID GLANDS						
SU22.3: Demonstrate and document the correct clinical examination of thyroid swellings and discuss the differential diagnosis and their management.						
Name of Activity	Date Completed (dd-mm-yyyy)	Attempt at activity First (F) Repeat (R) Remedial (Re)	Rating Below (B) Meets (M) Exceeds (E) Expectations	Decision of Faculty Complete (C) Repeat (R) Remedial (Re)	Initial of Faculty and Date	Feedback Received Initial of Learner

THYROID AND PARATHYROID GLANDS

Name of Activity	Date Completed (dd-mm-yyyy)	Attempt at activity First (F) Repeat (R) Remedial (Re)	Rating Below (B) Meets (M) Exceeds (E) Expectations	Decision of Faculty Complete (C) Repeat (R) Remedial (Re)	Initial of Faculty and Date	Feedback Received Initial of Learner

SU23: ADRENAL GLAND

ADRENAL GLAND						
Name of Activity	Date Completed (dd-mm-yyyy)	Attempt at activity First (F) Repeat (R) Remedial (Re)	Rating Below (B) Meets (M) Exceeds (E) Expectations	Decision of Faculty Complete (C) Repeat (R) Remedial (Re)	Initial of Faculty and Date	Feedback Received Initial of Learner

SU24: PANCREAS

PANCREAS						
Name of Activity	Date Completed (dd-mm-yyyy)	Attempt at activity First (F) Repeat (R) Remedial (Re)	Rating Below (B) Meets (M) Exceeds (E) Expectations	Decision of Faculty Complete (C) Repeat (R) Remedial (Re)	Initial of Faculty and Date	Feedback Received Initial of Learner

SU25: BREAST

BREAST						
SU25.5: Demonstrate the correct technique to palpate the breast for breast swelling in a mannequin or equivalent.						
Name of Activity	Date Completed (dd-mm-yyyy)	Attempt at activity First (F) Repeat (R) Remedial (Re)	Rating Below (B) Meets (M) Exceeds (E) Expectations	Decision of Faculty Complete (C) Repeat (R) Remedial (Re)	Initial of Faculty and Date	Feedback Received Initial of Learner

BREAST						
SU25.5: Demonstrate the correct technique to palpate the breast for breast swelling in a mannequin or equivalent.						
Name of Activity	*Date Completed (dd-mm-yyyy)*	*Attempt at activity First (F) Repeat (R) Remedial (Re)*	*Rating Below (B) Meets (M) Exceeds (E) Expectations*	*Decision of Faculty Complete (C) Repeat (R) Remedial (Re)*	*Initial of Faculty and Date*	*Feedback Received Initial of Learner*

		Attempt at activity First (F) Repeat (R) Remedial (Re)	Rating Below (B) Meets (M) Exceeds (E) Expectations	Decision of Faculty Complete (C) Repeat (R) Remedial (Re)	Initial of Faculty and Date	Feedback Received Initial of Learner
BREAST						
Name of Activity	Date Completed (dd-mm-yyyy)					

SU26: CARDIOTHORACIC SURGERY

CARDIOTHORACIC SURGERY						
Name of Activity	Date Completed (dd-mm-yyyy)	Attempt at activity First (F) Repeat (R) Remedial (Re)	Rating Below (B) Meets (M) Exceeds (E) Expectations	Decision of Faculty Complete (C) Repeat (R) Remedial (Re)	Initial of Faculty and Date	Feedback Received Initial of Learner

SU27: VASCULAR DISEASES

VASCULAR DISEASES

SU27.1: Describe the etiopathogenesis, clinical features, investigations and principles of treatment of occlusive arterial disease.

Name of Activity	Date Completed (dd-mm-yyyy)	Attempt at activity First (F) Repeat (R) Remedial (Re)	Rating Below (B) Meets (M) Exceeds (E) Expectations	Decision of Faculty Complete (C) Repeat (R) Remedial (Re)	Initial of Faculty and Date	Feedback Received Initial of Learner

VASCULAR DISEASES

SU27.2: Demonstrate the correct examination of the vascular system and enumerate and describe the investigation of vascular disease.

Name of Activity	Date Completed (dd-mm-yyyy)	Attempt at activity First (F) Repeat (R) Remedial (Re)	Rating Below (B) Meets (M) Exceeds (E) Expectations	Decision of Faculty Complete (C) Repeat (R) Remedial (Re)	Initial of Faculty and Date	Feedback Received Initial of Learner

VASCULAR DISEASES

SU27.8: Demonstrate the correct examination of the lymphatic system and venous system.

Name of Activity	Date Completed (dd-mm-yyyy)	Attempt at activity First (F) Repeat (R) Remedial (Re)	Rating Below (B) Meets (M) Exceeds (E) Expectations	Decision of Faculty Complete (C) Repeat (R) Remedial (Re)	Initial of Faculty and Date	Feedback Received Initial of Learner

VASCULAR DISEASES						
Name of Activity	Date Completed (dd-mm-yyyy)	Attempt at activity First (F) Repeat (R) Remedial (Re)	Rating Below (B) Meets (M) Exceeds (E) Expectations	Decision of Faculty Complete (C) Repeat (R) Remedial (Re)	Initial of Faculty and Date	Feedback Received Initial of Learner

SU28: ABDOMEN

ABDOMEN						
SU28.9: Demonstrate the correct technique of examination of a patient with disorders of the stomach.						
Name of Activity	Date Completed (dd-mm-yyyy)	Attempt at activity First (F) Repeat (R) Remedial (Re)	Rating Below (B) Meets (M) Exceeds (E) Expectations	Decision of Faculty Complete (C) Repeat (R) Remedial (Re)	Initial of Faculty and Date	Feedback Received Initial of Learner

ABDOMEN						
Name of Activity	Date Completed (dd-mm-yyyy)	Attempt at activity First (F) Repeat (R) Remedial (Re)	Rating Below (B) Meets (M) Exceeds (E) Expectations	Decision of Faculty Complete (C) Repeat (R) Remedial (Re)	Initial of Faculty and Date	Feedback Received Initial of Learner

ABDOMEN						
Name of Activity	Date Completed (dd-mm-yyyy)	Attempt at activity First (F) Repeat (R) Remedial (Re)	Rating Below (B) Meets (M) Exceeds (E) Expectations	Decision of Faculty Complete (C) Repeat (R) Remedial (Re)	Initial of Faculty and Date	Feedback Received Initial of Learner

ABDOMEN

Name of Activity	Date Completed (dd-mm-yyyy)	Attempt at activity First (F) Repeat (R) Remedial (Re)	Rating Below (B) Meets (M) Exceeds (E) Expectations	Decision of Faculty Complete (C) Repeat (R) Remedial (Re)	Initial of Faculty and Date	Feedback Received Initial of Learner

ABDOMEN						
Name of Activity	Date Completed (dd-mm-yyyy)	Attempt at activity First (F) Repeat (R) Remedial (Re)	Rating Below (B) Meets (M) Exceeds (E) Expectations	Decision of Faculty Complete (C) Repeat (R) Remedial (Re)	Initial of Faculty and Date	Feedback Received Initial of Learner

SU29: URINARY SYSTEM

URINARY SYSTEM

SU29.10: Demonstrate a digital rectal examination of the prostate in a mannequin or equivalent.

Name of Activity	Date Completed (dd-mm-yyyy)	Attempt at activity First (F) Repeat (R) Remedial (Re)	Rating Below (B) Meets (M) Exceeds (E) Expectations	Decision of Faculty Complete (C) Repeat (R) Remedial (Re)	Initial of Faculty and Date	Feedback Received Initial of Learner

URINARY SYSTEM						
Name of Activity	*Date Completed (dd-mm-yyyy)*	*Attempt at activity First (F) Repeat (R) Remedial (Re)*	*Rating Below (B) Meets (M) Exceeds (E) Expectations*	*Decision of Faculty Complete (C) Repeat (R) Remedial (Re)*	*Initial of Faculty and Date*	*Feedback Received Initial of Learner*

URINARY SYSTEM

Name of Activity	Date Completed (dd-mm-yyyy)	Attempt at activity First (F) Repeat (R) Remedial (Re)	Rating Below (B) Meets (M) Exceeds (E) Expectations	Decision of Faculty Complete (C) Repeat (R) Remedial (Re)	Initial of Faculty and Date	Feedback Received Initial of Learner

SU30: PENIS, TESTIS AND SCROTUM

PENIS, TESTIS AND SCROTUM						
Name of Activity	Date Completed (dd-mm-yyyy)	Attempt at activity First (F) Repeat (R) Remedial (Re)	Rating Below (B) Meets (M) Exceeds (E) Expectations	Decision of Faculty Complete (C) Repeat (R) Remedial (Re)	Initial of Faculty and Date	Feedback Received Initial of Learner

ORTHOPEDICS

TOPIC: SKELETAL TRAUMA						
OR1.6: Participate as a member in the team for closed reduction of shoulder dislocation/hip dislocation/knee dislocation.						
Name of Activity	Date Completed (dd-mm-yyyy)	Attempt at activity First (F) Repeat (R) Remedial (Re)	Rating Below (B) Meets (M) Exceeds (E) Expectations	Decision of Faculty Complete (C) Repeat (R) Remedial (Re)	Initial of Faculty and Date	Feedback Received Initial of Learner

Name of Activity	Date Completed (dd-mm-yyyy)	Attempt at activity First (F) Repeat (R) Remedial (Re)	Rating Below (B) Meets (M) Exceeds (E) Expectations	Decision of Faculty Complete (C) Repeat (R) Remedial (Re)	Initial of Faculty and Date	Feedback Received Initial of Learner

OR2: FRACTURES

TOPIC: FRACTURES						
OR2.3: Select, prescribe and communicate appropriate medications for relief of joint pain.						
Name of Activity	Date Completed (dd-mm-yyyy)	Attempt at activity First (F) Repeat (R) Remedial (Re)	Rating Below (B) Meets (M) Exceeds (E) Expectations	Decision of Faculty Complete (C) Repeat (R) Remedial (Re)	Initial of Faculty and Date	Feedback Received Initial of Learner

TOPIC: FRACTURES

OR2.15: Plan and interpret the investigations to diagnose complications of fractures like malunion, non-union, infection, compartmental syndrome.

Name of Activity	Date Completed (dd-mm-yyyy)	Attempt at activity First (F) Repeat (R) Remedial (Re)	Rating Below (B) Meets (M) Exceeds (E) Expectations	Decision of Faculty Complete (C) Repeat (R) Remedial (Re)	Initial of Faculty and Date	Feedback Received Initial of Learner

TOPIC: FRACTURES						
Name of Activity	Date Completed (dd-mm-yyyy)	Attempt at activity First (F) Repeat (R) Remedial (Re)	Rating Below (B) Meets (M) Exceeds (E) Expectations	Decision of Faculty Complete (C) Repeat (R) Remedial (Re)	Initial of Faculty and Date	Feedback Received Initial of Learner

		Attempt at activity First (F) Repeat (R) Remedial (Re)	Rating Below (B) Meets (M) Exceeds (E) Expectations	Decision of Faculty Complete (C) Repeat (R) Remedial (Re)	Initial of Faculty and Date	Feedback Received Initial of Learner
Name of Activity	Date Completed (dd-mm-yyyy)					

TOPIC: FRACTURES						
Name of Activity	*Date Completed (dd-mm-yyyy)*	*Attempt at activity First (F) Repeat (R) Remedial (Re)*	*Rating Below (B) Meets (M) Exceeds (E) Expectations*	*Decision of Faculty Complete (C) Repeat (R) Remedial (Re)*	*Initial of Faculty and Date*	*Feedback Received Initial of Learner*

▊ OR3: MUSCULOSKELETAL INFECTION

TOPIC: MUSCULOSKELETAL INFECTION						
OR3.2: Participate as a member in team for aspiration of joints under supervision.						
Name of Activity	Date Completed (dd-mm-yyyy)	Attempt at activity First (F) Repeat (R) Remedial (Re)	Rating Below (B) Meets (M) Exceeds (E) Expectations	Decision of Faculty Complete (C) Repeat (R) Remedial (Re)	Initial of Faculty and Date	Feedback Received Initial of Learner

TOPIC: MUSCULOSKELETAL INFECTION

OR3.3: Participate as a member in team for procedures like drainage of abscess, sequestrectomy/saucerisation and arthrotomy.

Name of Activity	Date Completed (dd-mm-yyyy)	Attempt at activity First (F) Repeat (R) Remedial (Re)	Rating Below (B) Meets (M) Exceeds (E) Expectations	Decision of Faculty Complete (C) Repeat (R) Remedial (Re)	Initial of Faculty and Date	Feedback Received Initial of Learner

OR4: SKELETAL TUBERCULOSIS

TOPIC: SKELETAL TUBERCULOSIS						
Name of Activity	Date Completed (dd-mm-yyyy)	Attempt at activity First (F) Repeat (R) Remedial (Re)	Rating Below (B) Meets (M) Exceeds (E) Expectations	Decision of Faculty Complete (C) Repeat (R) Remedial (Re)	Initial of Faculty and Date	Feedback Received Initial of Learner

OR5: RHEUMATOID ARTHRITIS AND ASSOCIATED INFLAMMATORY DISORDERS

TOPIC: RHEUMATOID ARTHRITIS AND ASSOCIATED INFLAMMATORY DISORDERS						
Name of Activity	Date Completed (dd-mm-yyyy)	Attempt at activity First (F) Repeat (R) Remedial (Re)	Rating Below (B) Meets (M) Exceeds (E) Expectations	Decision of Faculty Complete (C) Repeat (R) Remedial (Re)	Initial of Faculty and Date	Feedback Received Initial of Learner

OR6: DEGENERATIVE DISORDERS

TOPIC: DEGENERATIVE DISORDERS						
Name of Activity	Date Completed (dd-mm-yyyy)	Attempt at activity First (F) Repeat (R) Remedial (Re)	Rating Below (B) Meets (M) Exceeds (E) Expectations	Decision of Faculty Complete (C) Repeat (R) Remedial (Re)	Initial of Faculty and Date	Feedback Received Initial of Learner

OR7: METABOLIC BONE DISORDER

TOPIC: METABOLIC BONE DISORDER						
Name of Activity	Date Completed (dd-mm-yyyy)	Attempt at activity First (F) Repeat (R) Remedial (Re)	Rating Below (B) Meets (M) Exceeds (E) Expectations	Decision of Faculty Complete (C) Repeat (R) Remedial (Re)	Initial of Faculty and Date	Feedback Received Initial of Learner

OR8: POLIOMYELITIS

TOPIC: POLIOMYELITIS						
Name of Activity	Date Completed (dd-mm-yyyy)	Attempt at activity First (F) Repeat (R) Remedial (Re)	Rating Below (B) Meets (M) Exceeds (E) Expectations	Decision of Faculty Complete (C) Repeat (R) Remedial (Re)	Initial of Faculty and Date	Feedback Received Initial of Learner

OR9: CEREBRAL PALSY

TOPIC: CEREBRAL PALSY						
Name of Activity	Date Completed (dd-mm-yyyy)	Attempt at activity First (F) Repeat (R) Remedial (Re)	Rating Below (B) Meets (M) Exceeds (E) Expectations	Decision of Faculty Complete (C) Repeat (R) Remedial (Re)	Initial of Faculty and Date	Feedback Received Initial of Learner

OR10: BONE TUMOURS

TOPIC: BONE TUMOURS						
Name of Activity	Date Completed (dd-mm-yyyy)	Attempt at activity First (F) Repeat (R) Remedial (Re)	Rating Below (B) Meets (M) Exceeds (E) Expectations	Decision of Faculty Complete (C) Repeat (R) Remedial (Re)	Initial of Faculty and Date	Feedback Received Initial of Learner

OR11: PERIPHERAL NERVE INJURIES

TOPIC: PERIPHERAL NERVE INJURIES						
Name of Activity	Date Completed (dd-mm-yyyy)	Attempt at activity First (F) Repeat (R) Remedial (Re)	Rating Below (B) Meets (M) Exceeds (E) Expectations	Decision of Faculty Complete (C) Repeat (R) Remedial (Re)	Initial of Faculty and Date	Feedback Received Initial of Learner

OR12: CONGENITAL LESIONS

TOPIC: CONGENITAL LESIONS						
Name of Activity	Date Completed (dd-mm-yyyy)	Attempt at activity First (F) Repeat (R) Remedial (Re)	Rating Below (B) Meets (M) Exceeds (E) Expectations	Decision of Faculty Complete (C) Repeat (R) Remedial (Re)	Initial of Faculty and Date	Feedback Received Initial of Learner

OR13: PROCEDURAL SKILLS

TOPIC: PROCEDURAL SKILLS

OR13.1: Participate in a team for procedures in patients and demonstrating the ability to perform on mannequins/simulated patients in the following:

i. Above elbow plaster
ii. Below knee plaster
iii. Above knee plaster
iv. Thomas splint
v. Splinting for long bone fractures
vi. Strapping for shoulder and clavicle trauma

Name of Activity	Date Completed (dd-mm-yyyy)	Attempt at activity First (F) Repeat (R) Remedial (Re)	Rating Below (B) Meets (M) Exceeds (E) Expectations	Decision of Faculty Complete (C) Repeat (R) Remedial (Re)	Initial of Faculty and Date	Feedback Received Initial of Learner

TOPIC: PROCEDURAL SKILLS

OR13.2: Participate as a member in team for resuscitation of polytrauma victim by doing all of the following:
a. I.V. access central - peripheral
b. Bladder catheterization
c. Endotracheal intubation
d. Splintage

Name of Activity	Date Completed (dd-mm-yyyy)	Attempt at activity First (F) Repeat (R) Remedial (Re)	Rating Below (B) Meets (M) Exceeds (E) Expectations	Decision of Faculty Complete (C) Repeat (R) Remedial (Re)	Initial of Faculty and Date	Feedback Received Initial of Learner

OR14: COUNSELLING SKILLS

TOPIC: COUNSELLING SKILLS

OR14.1: Demonstrate the ability to counsel patients regarding prognosis in patients with various orthopedic illnesses like:
a. Fractures with disabilities b. Fractures that require prolonged bed stay
c. Bone tumours d. Congenital disabilities

Name of Activity	Date Completed (dd-mm-yyyy)	Attempt at activity First (F) Repeat (R) Remedial (Re)	Rating Below (B) Meets (M) Exceeds (E) Expectations	Decision of Faculty Complete (C) Repeat (R) Remedial (Re)	Initial of Faculty and Date	Feedback Received Initial of Learner

TOPIC: COUNSELING SKILLS

OR14.2: Demonstrate the ability to counsel patients to obtain consent for various orthopedic procedures like limp amputation, permanent fixations, etc.

Name of Activity	Date Completed (dd-mm-yyyy)	Attempt at activity First (F) Repeat (R) Remedial (Re)	Rating Below (B) Meets (M) Exceeds (E) Expectations	Decision of Faculty Complete (C) Repeat (R) Remedial (Re)	Initial of Faculty and Date	Feedback Received Initial of Learner

Name of Activity	Date Completed (dd-mm-yyyy)	Attempt at activity First (F) Repeat (R) Remedial (Re)	Rating Below (B) Meets (M) Exceeds (E) Expectations	Decision of Faculty Complete (C) Repeat (R) Remedial (Re)	Initial of Faculty and Date	Feedback Received Initial of Learner

TOPIC: COUNSELING SKILLS						
OR14.3: Demonstrate the ability to convince the patient for referral to a higher centre in various orthopedic illnesses, based on the detection of warning signals and need for sophisticated management.						
Name of Activity	Date Completed (dd-mm-yyyy)	Attempt at activity First (F) Repeat (R) Remedial (Re)	Rating Below (B) Meets (M) Exceeds (E) Expectations	Decision of Faculty Complete (C) Repeat (R) Remedial (Re)	Initial of Faculty and Date	Feedback Received Initial of Learner

AS2: CARDIOPULMONARY RESUSCITATION

TOPIC: CARDIOPULMONARY RESUSCITATION						
Name of Activity	Date Completed (dd-mm-yyyy)	Attempt at activity First (F) Repeat (R) Remedial (Re)	Rating Below (B) Meets (M) Exceeds (E) Expectations	Decision of Faculty Complete (C) Repeat (R) Remedial (Re)	Initial of Faculty and Date	Feedback Received Initial of Learner

AS3: PREOPERATIVE EVALUATION AND MEDICATION

TOPIC: PREOPERATIVE EVALUATION AND MEDICATION						
AS3.3: Demonstrate and document an appropriate clinical examination in a patient undergoing general surgery.						
Name of Activity	Date Completed (dd-mm-yyyy)	Attempt at activity First (F) Repeat (R) Remedial (Re)	Rating Below (B) Meets (M) Exceeds (E) Expectations	Decision of Faculty Complete (C) Repeat (R) Remedial (Re)	Initial of Faculty and Date	Feedback Received Initial of Learner

TOPIC: PREOPERATIVE EVALUATION AND MEDICATION

AS3.3: Demonstrate and document an appropriate clinical examination in a patient undergoing general surgery.

Name of Activity	Date Completed (dd-mm-yyyy)	Attempt at activity First (F) Repeat (R) Remedial (Re)	Rating Below (B) Meets (M) Exceeds (E) Expectations	Decision of Faculty Complete (C) Repeat (R) Remedial (Re)	Initial of Faculty and Date	Feedback Received Initial of Learner

AS4: GENERAL ANESTHESIA

TOPIC: GENERAL ANESTHESIA						
AS4.3: Observe and describe the principles and the practical aspects of induction and maintenance of anesthesia.						
Name of Activity	Date Completed (dd-mm-yyyy)	Attempt at activity First (F) Repeat (R) Remedial (Re)	Rating Below (B) Meets (M) Exceeds (E) Expectations	Decision of Faculty Complete (C) Repeat (R) Remedial (Re)	Initial of Faculty and Date	Feedback Received Initial of Learner

TOPIC: GENERAL ANESTHESIA

AS4.4: Observe and describe the principles and the steps/techniques in maintenance of vital organ functions in patients undergoing surgical procedures.

Name of Activity	Date Completed (dd-mm-yyyy)	Attempt at activity First (F) Repeat (R) Remedial (Re)	Rating Below (B) Meets (M) Exceeds (E) Expectations	Decision of Faculty Complete (C) Repeat (R) Remedial (Re)	Initial of Faculty and Date	Feedback Received Initial of Learner

TOPIC: GENERAL ANESTHESIA						

AS4.5: Observe and describe the principles and the steps/techniques in monitoring patients during anesthesia.
AS4.6: Observe and describe the principles and the steps/techniques involved in day care anesthesia.
AS4.7: Observe and describe the principles and the steps/techniques involved in anesthesia outside the operating room.

Name of Activity	Date Completed (dd-mm-yyyy)	Attempt at activity First (F) Repeat (R) Remedial (Re)	Rating Below (B) Meets (M) Exceeds (E) Expectations	Decision of Faculty Complete (C) Repeat (R) Remedial (Re)	Initial of Faculty and Date	Feedback Received Initial of Learner

TOPIC: GENERAL ANESTHESIA

AS4.5: Observe and describe the principles and the steps/techniques in monitoring patients during anesthesia.
AS4.6: Observe and describe the principles and the steps/techniques involved in day care anesthesia.
AS4.7: Observe and describe the principles and the steps/techniques involved in anesthesia outside the operating room.

Name of Activity	Date Completed (dd-mm-yyyy)	Attempt at activity First (F) Repeat (R) Remedial (Re)	Rating Below (B) Meets (M) Exceeds (E) Expectations	Decision of Faculty Complete (C) Repeat (R) Remedial (Re)	Initial of Faculty and Date	Feedback Received Initial of Learner

AS5: REGIONAL ANESTHESIA

TOPIC: REGIONAL ANESTHESIA						
AS5.3: Observe and describe the principles and steps/techniques involved in peripheral nerve blocks.						
Name of Activity	Date Completed (dd-mm-yyyy)	Attempt at activity First (F) Repeat (R) Remedial (Re)	Rating Below (B) Meets (M) Exceeds (E) Expectations	Decision of Faculty Complete (C) Repeat (R) Remedial (Re)	Initial of Faculty and Date	Feedback Received Initial of Learner

TOPIC: REGIONAL ANESTHESIA

AS5.4: Observe and describe the pharmacology and correct use of commonly used drugs and adjuvant agents in regional anesthesia.

Name of Activity	Date Completed (dd-mm-yyyy)	Attempt at activity First (F) Repeat (R) Remedial (Re)	Rating Below (B) Meets (M) Exceeds (E) Expectations	Decision of Faculty Complete (C) Repeat (R) Remedial (Re)	Initial of Faculty and Date	Feedback Received Initial of Learner

TOPIC: REGIONAL ANESTHESIA

AS5.5: Observe and describe the principles and steps/techniques involved in caudal epidural in adults and children.

Name of Activity	Date Completed (dd-mm-yyyy)	Attempt at activity First (F) Repeat (R) Remedial (Re)	Rating Below (B) Meets (M) Exceeds (E) Expectations	Decision of Faculty Complete (C) Repeat (R) Remedial (Re)	Initial of Faculty and Date	Feedback Received Initial of Learner

TOPIC: REGIONAL ANESTHESIA						
AS5.6: Observe and describe the principles and steps/techniques involved in common blocks used in surgery (including brachial plexus blocks).						
Name of Activity	Date Completed (dd-mm-yyyy)	Attempt at activity First (F) Repeat (R) Remedial (Re)	Rating Below (B) Meets (M) Exceeds (E) Expectations	Decision of Faculty Complete (C) Repeat (R) Remedial (Re)	Initial of Faculty and Date	Feedback Received Initial of Learner

AS6: POST-ANESTHESIA RECOVERY

TOPIC: POST-ANESTHESIA RECOVERY						
AS6.2: Observe and enumerate the contents of the crash cart and describe the equipment used in the recovery room.						
Name of Activity	Date Completed (dd-mm-yyyy)	Attempt at activity First (F) Repeat (R) Remedial (Re)	Rating Below (B) Meets (M) Exceeds (E) Expectations	Decision of Faculty Complete (C) Repeat (R) Remedial (Re)	Initial of Faculty and Date	Feedback Received Initial of Learner

TOPIC: POST-ANESTHESIA RECOVERY						
AS6.3: Describe the common complications encountered by patients in the recovery room, their recognition and principles of management.						
Name of Activity	Date Completed (dd-mm-yyyy)	Attempt at activity First (F) Repeat (R) Remedial (Re)	Rating Below (B) Meets (M) Exceeds (E) Expectations	Decision of Faculty Complete (C) Repeat (R) Remedial (Re)	Initial of Faculty and Date	Feedback Received Initial of Learner

AS7: INTENSIVE CARE MANAGEMENT

TOPIC: INTENSIVE CARE MANAGEMENT						
AS7.1: Visit, enumerate and describe the functions of an intensive care unit.						
Name of Activity	Date Completed (dd-mm-yyyy)	Attempt at activity First (F) Repeat (R) Remedial (Re)	Rating Below (B) Meets (M) Exceeds (E) Expectations	Decision of Faculty Complete (C) Repeat (R) Remedial (Re)	Initial of Faculty and Date	Feedback Received Initial of Learner

TOPIC: INTENSIVE CARE MANAGEMENT

AS7.3: Observe and describe the management of an unconscious patient.

Name of Activity	Date Completed (dd-mm-yyyy)	Attempt at activity First (F) Repeat (R) Remedial (Re)	Rating Below (B) Meets (M) Exceeds (E) Expectations	Decision of Faculty Complete (C) Repeat (R) Remedial (Re)	Initial of Faculty and Date	Feedback Received Initial of Learner

TOPIC: INTENSIVE CARE MANAGEMENT

AS7.4: Observe and describe the basic setup process of a ventilator.

Name of Activity	Date Completed (dd-mm-yyyy)	Attempt at activity First (F) Repeat (R) Remedial (Re)	Rating Below (B) Meets (M) Exceeds (E) Expectations	Decision of Faculty Complete (C) Repeat (R) Remedial (Re)	Initial of Faculty and Date	Feedback Received Initial of Learner

TOPIC: INTENSIVE CARE MANAGEMENT						
AS7.5: Observe and describe the principles of monitoring in an ICU.						
Name of Activity	*Date Completed (dd-mm-yyyy)*	*Attempt at activity* *First (F)* *Repeat (R)* *Remedial (Re)*	*Rating* *Below (B)* *Meets (M)* *Exceeds (E)* *Expectations*	*Decision of Faculty* *Complete (C)* *Repeat (R)* *Remedial (Re)*	*Initial of Faculty and Date*	*Feedback Received Initial of Learner*

AS8: PAIN AND ITS MANAGEMENT

TOPIC: PAIN AND ITS MANAGEMENT

AS8.2: Elicit and determine the level, quality and quantity of pain and its tolerance in patient or surrogate.

Name of Activity	Date Completed (dd-mm-yyyy)	Attempt at activity First (F) Repeat (R) Remedial (Re)	Rating Below (B) Meets (M) Exceeds (E) Expectations	Decision of Faculty Complete (C) Repeat (R) Remedial (Re)	Initial of Faculty and Date	Feedback Received Initial of Learner

AS9: FLUIDS

TOPIC: FLUIDS						
AS9.1: Establish intravenous access in a simulated environment.						
Name of Activity	Date Completed (dd-mm-yyyy)	Attempt at activity First (F) Repeat (R) Remedial (Re)	Rating Below (B) Meets (M) Exceeds (E) Expectations	Decision of Faculty Complete (C) Repeat (R) Remedial (Re)	Initial of Faculty and Date	Feedback Received Initial of Learner

TOPIC: FLUIDS

AS9.2: Establish central venous access in a simulated environment.

Name of Activity	Date Completed (dd-mm-yyyy)	Attempt at activity First (F) Repeat (R) Remedial (Re)	Rating Below (B) Meets (M) Exceeds (E) Expectations	Decision of Faculty Complete (C) Repeat (R) Remedial (Re)	Initial of Faculty and Date	Feedback Received Initial of Learner

AS10: PATIENT SAFETY

TOPIC: PATIENT SAFETY						
Name of Activity	Date Completed (dd-mm-yyyy)	Attempt at activity First (F) Repeat (R) Remedial (Re)	Rating Below (B) Meets (M) Exceeds (E) Expectations	Decision of Faculty Complete (C) Repeat (R) Remedial (Re)	Initial of Faculty and Date	Feedback Received Initial of Learner

RADIODIAGNOSIS

<table>
<tr><td colspan="7">TOPIC: RADIOLOGICAL INVESTIGATIONS AND RADIATION SAFETY</td></tr>
<tr>
<td>Name of Activity</td>
<td>Date Completed (dd-mm-yyyy)</td>
<td>Attempt at activity
First (F)
Repeat (R)
Remedial (Re)</td>
<td>Rating
Below (B)
Meets (M)
Exceeds (E)
Expectations</td>
<td>Decision of Faculty
Complete (C)
Repeat (R)
Remedial (Re)</td>
<td>Initial of Faculty and Date</td>
<td>Feedback Received
Initial of Learner</td>
</tr>
<tr><td></td><td></td><td></td><td></td><td></td><td></td><td></td></tr>
<tr><td></td><td></td><td></td><td></td><td></td><td></td><td></td></tr>
<tr><td></td><td></td><td></td><td></td><td></td><td></td><td></td></tr>
<tr><td></td><td></td><td></td><td></td><td></td><td></td><td></td></tr>
</table>

Name of Activity	Date Completed (dd-mm-yyyy)	Attempt at activity First (F) Repeat (R) Remedial (Re)	Rating Below (B) Meets (M) Exceeds (E) Expectations	Decision of Faculty Complete (C) Repeat (R) Remedial (Re)	Initial of Faculty and Date	Feedback Received Initial of Learner

4.1: THE FOUNDATIONS OF COMMUNICATION

1. Demonstrate ability to communicate to patients in a patient, respectful, nonthreatening, non-judgmental and empathetic manner.

Name of Activity	Date Completed (dd-mm-yyyy)	Attempt at activity First (F) Repeat (R) Remedial (Re)	Rating Below (B) Meets (M) Exceeds (E) Expectations	Decision of Faculty Complete (C) Repeat (R) Remedial (Re)	Initial of Faculty and Date	Feedback Received Initial of Learner

4.1: THE FOUNDATIONS OF COMMUNICATION

2. Communicate diagnostic and therapeutic options to patient and family in a simulated environment.

Name of Activity	Date Completed (dd-mm-yyyy)	Attempt at activity First (F) Repeat (R) Remedial (Re)	Rating Below (B) Meets (M) Exceeds (E) Expectations	Decision of Faculty Complete (C) Repeat (R) Remedial (Re)	Initial of Faculty and Date	Feedback Received Initial of Learner

4.2: CASE STUDIES IN MEDICOLEGAL AND ETHICAL SITUATIONS

Identify, discuss and defend medicolegal, socioeconomic and ethical issues as it pertains to abortion/medical termination of pregnancy and reproductive rights.

Name of Activity	Date Completed (dd-mm-yyyy)	Attempt at activity First (F) Repeat (R) Remedial (Re)	Rating Below (B) Meets (M) Exceeds (E) Expectations	Decision of Faculty Complete (C) Repeat (R) Remedial (Re)	Initial of Faculty and Date	Feedback Received Initial of Learner

4.3: CASE STUDIES IN MEDICOLEGAL AND ETHICAL SITUATIONS

Identify and discuss medicolegal, socioeconomic and ethical issues as it pertains to organ donation.

Name of Activity	Date Completed (dd-mm-yyyy)	Attempt at activity First (F) Repeat (R) Remedial (Re)	Rating Below (B) Meets (M) Exceeds (E) Expectations	Decision of Faculty Complete (C) Repeat (R) Remedial (Re)	Initial of Faculty and Date	Feedback Received Initial of Learner

4.4: CASE STUDIES IN ETHICS EMPATHY AND THE DOCTOR-PATIENT RELATIONSHIP

1. Demonstrate empathy in patient encounters.

Name of Activity	Date Completed (dd-mm-yyyy)	Attempt at activity First (F) Repeat (R) Remedial (Re)	Rating Below (B) Meets (M) Exceeds (E) Expectations	Decision of Faculty Complete (C) Repeat (R) Remedial (Re)	Initial of Faculty and Date	Feedback Received Initial of Learner

4.4: CASE STUDIES IN ETHICS EMPATHY AND THE DOCTOR-PATIENT RELATIONSHIP

2. Communicate care options to patient and family with a terminal illness in a simulated environment.

Name of Activity	Date Completed (dd-mm-yyyy)	Attempt at activity First (F) Repeat (R) Remedial (Re)	Rating Below (B) Meets (M) Exceeds (E) Expectations	Decision of Faculty Complete (C) Repeat (R) Remedial (Re)	Initial of Faculty and Date	Feedback Received Initial of Learner

4.5: CASE STUDIES IN ETHICS: THE DOCTOR-INDUSTRY RELATIONSHIP

Identify and discuss and defend medicolegal, sociocultural, professional and ethical issues in physician-industry relationships.

Name of Activity	Date Completed (dd-mm-yyyy)	Attempt at activity First (F) Repeat (R) Remedial (Re)	Rating Below (B) Meets (M) Exceeds (E) Expectations	Decision of Faculty Complete (C) Repeat (R) Remedial (Re)	Initial of Faculty and Date	Feedback Received Initial of Learner

4.6: CASE STUDIES IN ETHICS: THE DOCTOR-INDUSTRY RELATIONSHIP

Identify conflicts of interest in patient care and professional relationships and describe the correct response to these conflicts.

Name of Activity	Date Completed (dd-mm-yyyy)	Attempt at activity First (F) Repeat (R) Remedial (Re)	Rating Below (B) Meets (M) Exceeds (E) Expectations	Decision of Faculty Complete (C) Repeat (R) Remedial (Re)	Initial of Faculty and Date	Feedback Received Initial of Learner

4.7: CASE STUDIES IN ETHICS AND PATIENT AUTONOMY

Identify conflicts of interest in patient care and professional relationships and describe the correct response to these conflicts.

Name of Activity	Date Completed (dd-mm-yyyy)	Attempt at activity First (F) Repeat (R) Remedial (Re)	Rating Below (B) Meets (M) Exceeds (E) Expectations	Decision of Faculty Complete (C) Repeat (R) Remedial (Re)	Initial of Faculty and Date	Feedback Received Initial of Learner

4.8: DEALING WITH DEATH

1. Identify conflicts of interest in patient care and professional relationships and describe the correct response to these conflicts.

Name of Activity	Date Completed (dd-mm-yyyy)	Attempt at activity First (F) Repeat (R) Remedial (Re)	Rating Below (B) Meets (M) Exceeds (E) Expectations	Decision of Faculty Complete (C) Repeat (R) Remedial (Re)	Initial of Faculty and Date	Feedback Received Initial of Learner

4.8: DEALING WITH DEATH

2. Demonstrate empathy to patient and family with a terminal illness in a simulated environment.

Name of Activity	Date Completed (dd-mm-yyyy)	Attempt at activity First (F) Repeat (R) Remedial (Re)	Rating Below (B) Meets (M) Exceeds (E) Expectations	Decision of Faculty Complete (C) Repeat (R) Remedial (Re)	Initial of Faculty and Date	Feedback Received Initial of Learner

4.9: MEDICAL NEGLIGENCE

1. Identify, discuss and defend medicolegal, sociocultural, professional and ethical issues pertaining to medical negligence.

Name of Activity	Date Completed (dd-mm-yyyy)	Attempt at activity First (F) Repeat (R) Remedial (Re)	Rating Below (B) Meets (M) Exceeds (E) Expectations	Decision of Faculty Complete (C) Repeat (R) Remedial (Re)	Initial of Faculty and Date	Feedback Received Initial of Learner

4.9: MEDICAL NEGLIGENCE

2. Identify, discuss and defend medicolegal, sociocultural, professional and ethical issues pertaining to malpractice.

Name of Activity	Date Completed (dd-mm-yyyy)	Attempt at activity First (F) Repeat (R) Remedial (Re)	Rating Below (B) Meets (M) Exceeds (E) Expectations	Decision of Faculty Complete (C) Repeat (R) Remedial (Re)	Initial of Faculty and Date	Feedback Received Initial of Learner

SURGICAL PROCEDURE LOGBOOK

	SURGICAL PROCEDURE LOGBOOK					
Date	Name of Procedure	Role Independently Performed (IP) Performed under Supervision (SP) Assisted (A)	Rating Below (B) Meets (M) Exceeds (E) Expectations	Final Diagnosis	Initial of Faculty and Date	Feedback Received Initial of Learner

SURGICAL PROCEDURE LOGBOOK						
Date	Name of Procedure	Role Independently Performed (IP) Performed under Supervision (SP) Assisted (A)	Rating Below (B) Meets (M) Exceeds (E) Expectations	Final Diagnosis	Initial of Faculty and Date	Feedback Received Initial of Learner

		Role Independently Performed (IP) Performed under Supervision (SP) Assisted (A)	Rating Below (B) Meets (M) Exceeds (E) Expectations	Final Diagnosis	Initial of Faculty and Date	Feedback Received Initial of Learner
Date	Name of Procedure					

SURGICAL PROCEDURE LOGBOOK

Date	Name of Procedure	Role Independently Performed (IP) Performed under Supervision (SP) Assisted (A)	Rating Below (B) Meets (M) Exceeds (E) Expectations	Final Diagnosis	Initial of Faculty and Date	Feedback Received Initial of Learner

		Role Independently Performed (IP) Performed under Supervision (SP) Assisted (A)	Rating Below (B) Meets (M) Exceeds (E) Expectations			Feedback Received
SURGICAL PROCEDURE LOGBOOK						
Date	Name of Procedure			Final Diagnosis	Initial of Faculty and Date	Initial of Learner

		SURGICAL PROCEDURE LOGBOOK				
Date	Name of Procedure	Role Independently Performed (IP) Performed under Supervision (SP) Assisted (A)	Rating Below (B) Meets (M) Exceeds (E) Expectations	Final Diagnosis	Initial of Faculty and Date	Feedback Received Initial of Learner

		Role Independently Performed (IP) Performed under Supervision (SP) Assisted (A)	Rating Below (B) Meets (M) Exceeds (E) Expectations			Feedback Received
Date	Name of Procedure			Final Diagnosis	Initial of Faculty and Date	Initial of Learner

SURGICAL PROCEDURE LOGBOOK

Date	Name of Procedure	Role Independently Performed (IP) Performed under Supervision (SP) Assisted (A)	Rating Below (B) Meets (M) Exceeds (E) Expectations	Final Diagnosis	Initial of Faculty and Date	Feedback Received Initial of Learner

SURGICAL PROCEDURE LOGBOOK						
Date	Name of Procedure	Role Independently Performed (IP) Performed under Supervision (SP) Assisted (A)	Rating Below (B) Meets (M) Exceeds (E) Expectations	Final Diagnosis	Initial of Faculty and Date	Feedback Received Initial of Learner

		SURGICAL PROCEDURE LOGBOOK				
Date	Name of Procedure	Role Independently Performed (IP) Performed under Supervision (SP) Assisted (A)	Rating Below (B) Meets (M) Exceeds (E) Expectations	Final Diagnosis	Initial of Faculty and Date	Feedback Received Initial of Learner

		Role Independently Performed (IP) Performed under Supervision (SP) Assisted (A)	Rating Below (B) Meets (M) Exceeds (E) Expectations			
Date	Name of Procedure			Final Diagnosis	Initial of Faculty and Date	Feedback Received Initial of Learner

		Number performed			Initial of Faculty and Date	Feedback Received Initial of Learner
		Independently Performed (IP)	Performed under Supervision (SP)	Assisted (A)		
System	Name of Procedure					

SURGICAL PROCEDURE LOGBOOK-MASTERLIST

SURGICAL PROCEDURE LOGBOOK-MASTERLIST						
		Number performed			Initial of Faculty and Date	Feedback Received Initial of Learner
System	Name of Procedure	Independently Performed (IP)	Performed under Supervision (SP)	Assisted (A)		

SURGICAL PROCEDURE LOGBOOK-MASTERLIST

System	Name of Procedure	Number performed			Initial of Faculty and Date	Feedback Received Initial of Learner
		Independently Performed (IP)	Performed under Supervision (SP)	Assisted (A)		

SURGICAL PROCEDURE LOGBOOK-MASTERLIST						
		Number performed			Initial of Faculty and Date	Feedback Received Initial of Learner
System	Name of Procedure	Independently Performed (IP)	Performed under Supervision (SP)	Assisted (A)		

SURGICAL PROCEDURE LOGBOOK-MASTERLIST

| System | Name of Procedure | Number performed | | | Initial of Faculty and Date | Feedback Received Initial of Learner |
		Independently Performed (IP)	Performed under Supervision (SP)	Assisted (A)		

SURGICAL PROCEDURE LOGBOOK-MASTERLIST						
		Number performed			Initial of Faculty and Date	Feedback Received Initial of Learner
System	Name of Procedure	Independently Performed (IP)	Performed under Supervision (SP)	Assisted (A)		

CASE PRESENTED-MASTERLIST			
System	Case-diagnosis (provisional/final)	Initial of faculty and date	Feedback received Initial of Learner

CASE PRESENTED-MASTERLIST			
System	Case-diagnosis (provisional/final)	Initial of faculty and date	Feedback received Initial of Learner

CASE PRESENTED-MASTERLIST			
System	Case-diagnosis (provisional/final)	Initial of faculty and date	Feedback received Initial of Learner
System	Case-diagnosis (provisional/final)	Initial of faculty and date	Feedback received Initial of Learner

CASE PRESENTED-MASTERLIST			
System	Case-diagnosis (provisional/final)	Initial of faculty and date	Feedback received Initial of Learner

CASE PRESENTED-MASTERLIST			
System	Case-diagnosis (provisional/final)	Initial of faculty and date	Feedback received Initial of Learner

CASE PRESENTED-MASTERLIST			
System	Case-diagnosis (provisional/final)	Initial of faculty and date	Feedback received Initial of Learner

ASSESSMENT PERFORMA

I _________________________________, after having assessed _____________________ thoroughly ____________ am confident in certifying him/her as below.

1.	Proficiency	
2.	Competency for performing independently	
3.	Competency of assisting in procedures	
4.	Research aptitude	
5.	Participation in discussion	
6.	Initiative	
7.	Attitude	
8.	Responsibility	
9.	Punctuality	
10.	Behaviour with colleagues, nursing staffs and paramedicals	
11.	Overall score	

Remarks:

Signature _________________________________

Name, designation and stamp of Certifying Faculty _________________________________

ASSESSMENT PERFORMA

I _________________________________, after having assessed _________________________ thoroughly ____________ am confident in certifying him/her as below.

1.	Proficiency	
2.	Competency for performing independently	
3.	Competency of assisting in procedures	
4.	Research aptitude	
5.	Participation in discussion	
6.	Initiative	
7.	Attitude	
8.	Responsibility	
9.	Punctuality	
10.	Behaviour with colleagues, nursing staffs and paramedicals	
11.	Overall score	

Remarks:

Signature _________________________________

Name, designation and stamp of Certifying Faculty _________________

ASSESSMENT PERFORMA

I _______________________________, after having assessed _____________________ thoroughly ___________ am confident in certifying him/her as below.

1.	Proficiency	
2.	Competency for performing independently	
3.	Competency of assisting in procedures	
4.	Research aptitude	
5.	Participation in discussion	
6.	Initiative	
7.	Attitude	
8.	Responsibility	
9.	Punctuality	
10.	Behaviour with colleagues, nursing staffs and paramedicals	
11.	Overall Score	

Remarks:

Signature _______________________________

Name, designation and stamp of Certifying Faculty _______________________

ASSESSMENT PERFORMA

I _________________________________, after having assessed _______________________ thoroughly ____________ am confident in certifying him/her as below.

1.	Proficiency	
2.	Competency for performing independently	
3.	Competency of assisting in procedures	
4.	Research aptitude	
5.	Participation in discussion	
6.	Initiative	
7.	Attitude	
8.	Responsibility	
9.	Punctuality	
10.	Behaviour with colleagues, nursing staffs and paramedicals	
11.	Overall Score	

Remarks:

Signature _________________________________

Name, designation and stamp of Certifying Faculty _________________

ASSESSMENT PERFORMA

I ___________________________________, after having assessed ______________________________ thoroughly _______________
am confident in certifying him/her as below.

1.	Proficiency	
2.	Competency for performing independently	
3.	Competency of assisting in procedures	
4.	Research aptitude	
5.	Participation in discussion	
6.	Initiative	
7.	Attitude	
8.	Responsibility	
9.	Punctuality	
10.	Behaviour with colleagues, nursing staffs and paramedicals	
11.	Overall Score	

Remarks:

Signature _____________________________________

Name, designation and stamp of Certifying Faculty ____________________

ASSESSMENT PERFORMA

I _________________________________, after having assessed _____________________________ thoroughly _____________ am confident in certifying him/her as below.

1.	Proficiency	
2.	Competency for performing independently	
3.	Competency of assisting in procedures	
4.	Research aptitude	
5.	Participation in discussion	
6.	Initiative	
7.	Attitude	
8.	Responsibility	
9.	Punctuality	
10.	Behaviour with colleagues, nursing staffs and paramedicals	
11.	Overall Score	

Remarks:

Signature ___________________________________

Name, designation and stamp of Certifying Faculty ___________________

ASSESSMENT PERFORMA

I _________________________________, after having assessed _____________________________ thoroughly _____________ am confident in certifying him/her as below.

1.	Proficiency	
2.	Competency for performing independently	
3.	Competency of assisting in procedures	
4.	Research aptitude	
5.	Participation in discussion	
6.	Initiative	
7.	Attitude	
8.	Responsibility	
9.	Punctuality	
10.	Behaviour with colleagues, nursing staffs and paramedicals	
11.	Overall Score	

Remarks:

Signature _________________________________

Name, designation and stamp of Certifying Faculty _________________

ASSESSMENT PERFORMA

I _________________________________, after having assessed _______________________ thoroughly ____________ am confident in certifying him/her as below.

1.	Proficiency	
2.	Competency for performing independently	
3.	Competency of assisting in procedures	
4.	Research aptitude	
5.	Participation in discussion	
6.	Initiative	
7.	Attitude	
8.	Responsibility	
9.	Punctuality	
10.	Behaviour with colleagues, nursing staffs and paramedicals	
11.	Overall Score	

Remarks:

Signature ___________________________________

Name, designation and stamp of Certifying Faculty ___________________

ASSESSMENT PERFORMA

I _________________________________, after having assessed _______________________ thoroughly _____________ am confident in certifying him/her as below.

1.	Proficiency	
2.	Competency for performing independently	
3.	Competency of assisting in procedures	
4.	Research aptitude	
5.	Participation in discussion	
6.	Initiative	
7.	Attitude	
8.	Responsibility	
9.	Punctuality	
10.	Behaviour with colleagues, nursing staffs and paramedicals	
11.	Overall Score	

Remarks:

Signature _______________________________

Name, designation and stamp of Certifying Faculty _______________

CASE RECORD

Case Number:　　　　　　　　　　　　　　Patient's Hospital ID__________

Date:　　　　　　　　　　　　　　　　　Ward ______ Unit Incharge ______________

Name _________________________ Age _________ Sex _________
Occupation_________________________________
Address ____
Date of admission ____

Presenting complaints:

History of present illness:

Past history:

Personal history:

Treatment history:

Family history:

Menstrual history:

Obstetric history:

Socioeconomic history:

Any other:

General physical examination:
GCS:
Nutritional status:
Performance scale (Kamofsky performance states, ECOG):
Blood pressure:
Pulse:
Respiratory rate:
Temperature:
Pallor ___ Icterus ___ Clubbing ____Cyanosis ____ Oedema ______
Lymphadenopathy: Cervical _______
                 Axillary _______
                 Inguinal _______
Other significant findings:

Systemic examination:
Respiratory system:

Cardiovascular system:

Nervous system:

Abdomen:

Local examination of _____________ (name the system)

Inspection:

Palpation:

Percussion:

Auscultation:

Provisional diagnosis:

Differential diagnosis:
Specific investigations and their relevance to the condition:
1. For confirmation of diagnosis

2. For determining extent of disease (if applicable)

Management:

Operative findings:

Pathology report:

Final diagnosis:

Diagrammatic Representation of Findings

Signature of Student _______________

Signature of Assessor _______________

CASE RECORD

Case Number: **Patient's Hospital ID**_________

Date: **Ward** ______ **Unit Incharge** _____________

Name ______________________________ Age __________ Sex __________

Occupation____________________________________

Address ____

Date of admission ____

Presenting complaints:

History of present illness:

Past history:

Personal history:

Treatment history:

Family history:

Menstrual history:

Obstetric history:

Socio-economic history:

Any other:

General physical examination:
GCS:
Nutritional Status
Performance scale (Kamofsky performance states, ECOG):
Blood pressure:
Pulse:
Respiratory rate:
Temperature:
Pallor ___ Icterus ___ Clubbing ____Cyanosis ____ Oedema ______
Lymphadenopathy: Cervical _______
　　　　　　　　　　Axillary _______
　　　　　　　　　　Inguinal _______
Other significant findings:

Systemic examination:
Respiratory system:

Cardiovascular system:

Nervous system:

Abdomen:

Local examination of _____________ (name the system)

Inspection:

Palpation:

Percussion:

Auscultation:

<table><tr><td>

Diagrammatic Representation of Findings

</td></tr></table>

Provisional diagnosis:

Differential diagnosis:
Specific investigations and their relevance to the condition:
1. **For confirmation of diagnosis**

2. **For determining extent of disease (if applicable)**

Management:

Operative findings:

Pathology report:

Final Diagnosis:

Signature of Student ____________

Signature of Assessor ______________

CASE RECORD

Case Number: **Patient's Hospital ID**___________

Date: **Ward** _______ **Unit Incharge** _______________

Name _________________________________ Age ___________ Sex ___________
Occupation____
Address ____
Date of admission ____

Presenting complaints:

History of present illness:

Past history:

Personal history:

Treatment history:

Family history:

Menstrual history:

Obstetric history:

Socio-economic history:

Any other:

General physical examination:
GCS:
Nutritional Status
Performance scale (Kamofsky performance states, ECOG):
Blood pressure:
Pulse:
Respiratory rate:
Temperature:
Pallor ___ Icterus ___ Clubbing ____Cyanosis ____ Oedema ______
Lymphadenopathy: Cervical _______
                            Axillary _______
                            Inguinal _______
Other significant findings:

Systemic examination:
Respiratory system:

Cardiovascular system:

Nervous system:

Abdomen:

Local examination of _____________ (name the system)

Inspection:

Palpation:

Percussion:

Auscultation:

Provisional diagnosis:

Differential diagnosis:
Specific investigations and their relevance to the condition:
1. For confirmation of diagnosis

2. For determining extent of disease (if applicable)

Management:

Operative findings:

Pathology report:

Final diagnosis:

Diagrammatic Representation of Findings

Signature of Student ______________

Signature of Assessor ______________

CASE RECORD

Case Number: **Patient's Hospital ID**__________

Date: **Ward** ______ **Unit Incharge** _____________

Name _________________________________ Age __________ Sex __________

Occupation____

Address ____

Date of admission ____

Presenting complaints:

History of present illness:

Past history:

Personal history:

Treatment history:

Family history:

Menstrual history:

Obstetric history:

Socioeconomic history:

Any other:

General physical examination:
GCS:
Nutritional Status
Performance scale (Kamofsky performance states, ECOG):
Blood pressure:
Pulse:
Respiratory rate:
Temperature:
Pallor ___ Icterus ___ Clubbing ____Cyanosis ____ Oedema ______
Lymphadenopathy: Cervical _______
                 Axillary _______
                 Inguinal _______
Other significant findings:

Systemic examination:
Respiratory system:

Cardiovascular system:

Nervous system:

Abdomen:

Local examination of _____________ (name the system)

Inspection:

Palpation:

Percussion:

Auscultation:

Diagrammatic Representation of Findings

Provisional diagnosis:

Differential diagnosis:
Specific investigations and their relevance to the condition:
1. For confirmation of diagnosis

2. For determining extent of disease (if applicable)

Management:

Operative findings:

Pathology report:

Final diagnosis:

Signature of Student ____________

Signature of Assessor ______________

CASE RECORD

Case Number:

Patient's Hospital ID__________

Date:

Ward ______ **Unit Incharge** _____________

Name ________________________________ Age ___________ Sex ___________
Occupation____
Address ____
Date of admission ____

Presenting complaints:

History of present illness:

Past history:

Personal history:

Treatment history:

Family history:

Menstrual history:

Obstetric history:

Socioeconomic history:

Any other:

General physical examination:
GCS:
Nutritional Status
Performance scale (Kamofsky performance states, ECOG):
Blood pressure:
Pulse:
Respiratory rate:
Temperature:
Pallor ___ Icterus ___ Clubbing ___ Cyanosis ___ Oedema ______
Lymphadenopathy: Cervical _______
                    Axillary _______
                    Inguinal _______
Other significant findings:

Systemic examination:
Respiratory system:

Cardiovascular system:

Nervous system:

Abdomen:

Local examination of ______________ (name the system)

Inspection:

Palpation:

Percussion:

Auscultation:

Provisional diagnosis:

Differential diagnosis:
Specific investigations and their relevance to the condition:
1. For confirmation of diagnosis

2. For determining extent of disease (if applicable)

Management:

Operative findings:

Pathology report:

Final diagnosis:

Diagrammatic Representation of Findings

Signature of Student ________________

Signature of Assessor ________________

CASE RECORD

Case Number:

Date:

Patient's Hospital ID__________

Ward ______ Unit Incharge ____________

Name ________________________ Age __________ Sex __________
Occupation_____________________________________
Address ____
Date of admission ____

Presenting complaints:

History of present illness:

Past history:

Personal history:

Treatment history:

Family history:

Menstrual history:

Obstetric history:

Socioeconomic history:

Any other:

General physical examination:
GCS:
Nutritional Status
Performance scale (Kamofsky performance states, ECOG):
Blood pressure:
Pulse:
Respiratory rate:
Temperature:
Pallor ___ Icterus ___ Clubbing ____Cyanosis ____ Oedema ______
Lymphadenopathy: Cervical _______
                 Axillary _______
                 Inguinal _______
Other significant findings:

Systemic examination:
Respiratory system:

Cardiovascular system:

Nervous system:

Abdomen:

Local examination of _____________ (name the system)

Inspection:

Palpation:

Percussion:

Auscultation:

Provisional diagnosis:

Differential diagnosis:
Specific investigations and their relevance to the condition:
1. For confirmation of diagnosis

2. For determining extent of disease (if applicable)

Management:

Operative findings:

Pathology report:

Final Diagnosis:

Diagrammatic Representation of Findings

Signature of Student ________________

Signature of Assessor ________________

CASE RECORD

Case Number: **Patient's Hospital ID**__________

Date: **Ward** ______ **Unit Incharge** _____________

Name ___________________________ Age __________ Sex __________
Occupation____
Address ____
Date of admission ____

Presenting complaints:

History of present illness:

Past history:

Personal history:

Treatment history:

Family history:

Menstrual history:

Obstetric history:

Socioeconomic history:

Any other:

General physical examination:
GCS:
Nutritional Status
Performance scale (Kamofsky performance states, ECOG):
Blood pressure:
Pulse:
Respiratory rate:
Temperature:
Pallor ___ Icterus ___ Clubbing ____Cyanosis ____ Oedema ______
Lymphadenopathy: Cervical _______
                 Axillary _______
                 Inguinal _______
Other significant findings:

Systemic examination:
Respiratory system:

Cardiovascular system:

Nervous system:

Abdomen:

Local examination of _____________ (name the system)

Inspection:

Palpation:

Percussion:

Auscultation:

Diagrammatic Representation of Findings

Provisional diagnosis:

Differential diagnosis:
Specific investigations and their relevance to the condition:
1. For confirmation of diagnosis

2. For determining extent of disease (if applicable)

Management:

Operative findings:

Pathology report:

Final diagnosis:

Signature of Student ___________

Signature of Assessor ___________

CASE RECORD

Case Number: **Patient's Hospital ID**___________

Date: **Ward** _______ **Unit Incharge** _______________

Name ________________________________ Age ___________ Sex ____________
Occupation____
Address ____
Date of admission ____

Presenting complaints:

History of present illness:

Past history:

Personal history:

Treatment history:

Family history:

Menstrual history:

Obstetric history:

Socioeconomic history:

Any other:

General physical examination:
GCS:
Nutritional Status
Performance scale (Kamofsky performance states, ECOG):
Blood pressure:
Pulse:
Respiratory rate:
Temperature:
Pallor ___ Icterus ___ Clubbing ___Cyanosis ____ Oedema ______
Lymphadenopathy: Cervical _______
                  Axillary _______
                  Inguinal _______
Other significant findings:

Systemic examination:
Respiratory system:

Cardiovascular system:

Nervous system:

Abdomen:

Local examination of _____________ (name the system)

Inspection:

Palpation:

Percussion:

Auscultation:

Diagrammatic Representation of Findings

Provisional diagnosis:

Differential diagnosis:
Specific investigations and their relevance to the condition:
1. **For confirmation of diagnosis**

2. **For determining extent of disease (if applicable)**

Management:

Operative findings:

Pathology report:

Final diagnosis:

Signature of Student ____________

Signature of Assessor ______________

CASE RECORD

Case Number:

Patient's Hospital ID__________

Date:

Ward ______ Unit Incharge ______________

Name ________________________________ Age ___________ Sex ___________
Occupation____
Address ____
Date of admission ____

Presenting complaints:

History of present illness:

Past history:

Personal history:

Treatment history:

Family history:

Menstrual history:

Obstetric history:

Socioeconomic history:

Any other:

General physical examination:
GCS:
Nutritional Status
Performance scale (Kamofsky performance states, ECOG):
Blood pressure:
Pulse:
Respiratory rate:
Temperature:
Pallor ___ Icterus ___ Clubbing ____Cyanosis ____ Oedema ______
Lymphadenopathy: Cervical ______
                 Axillary ______
                 Inguinal ______
Other significant findings:

Systemic examination:
Respiratory system:

Cardiovascular system:

Nervous system:

Abdomen:

Local examination of ____________ (name the system)

Inspection:

Palpation:

Percussion:

Auscultation:

Provisional diagnosis:

Differential diagnosis:
Specific investigations and their relevance to the condition:
1. **For confirmation of diagnosis**

2. **For determining extent of disease (if applicable)**

Management:

Operative findings:

Pathology report:

Final diagnosis:

Diagrammatic Representation of Findings

Signature of Student _______________

Signature of Assessor _______________

CASE RECORD

Case Number:

Date:

Patient's Hospital ID___________

Ward ______ **Unit Incharge** _______________

Name _________________________________ Age ___________ Sex ___________
Occupation____
Address ____
Date of admission ____

Presenting complaints:

History of present illness:

Past history:

Personal history:

Treatment history:

Family history:

Menstrual history:

Obstetric history:

Socioeconomic history:

Any other:

General physical examination:
GCS:
Nutritional Status
Performance scale (Kamofsky performance states, ECOG):
Blood pressure:
Pulse:
Respiratory rate:
Temperature:
Pallor ___ Icterus ___ Clubbing ____Cyanosis ____ Oedema ______
Lymphadenopathy: Cervical _______
                  Axillary _______
                  Inguinal _______
Other significant findings:

Systemic examination:
Respiratory system:

Cardiovascular system:

Nervous system:

Abdomen:

Local examination of _____________ (name the system)

Inspection:

Palpation:

Percussion:

Auscultation:

<table><tr><td>Diagrammatic Representation of Findings</td></tr></table>

Provisional diagnosis:

Differential diagnosis:
Specific investigations and their relevance to the condition:
1. **For confirmation of diagnosis**

2. **For determining extent of disease (if applicable)**

Management:

Operative findings:

Pathology report:

Final diagnosis:

Signature of Student _____________

Signature of Assessor _______________

ACADEMIC PRESENTATIONS

Date	Type Journal Club/Seminar/Clinical Case/ Audit/Other	Title of Procedure	Rating Below (B) Meets (M) Exceeds (E) Expectations	Initial of Faculty and Date	Feedback Received Initial of Learner

ACADEMIC PRESENTATIONS

Date	Type Journal Club/Seminar/Clinical Case/Audit/Other	Title of Procedure	Rating Below (B) Meets (M) Exceeds (E) Expectations	Initial of Faculty and Date	Feedback Received Initial of Learner

ACADEMIC PRESENTATIONS

Date	Type Journal Club/Seminar/Clinical Case/ Audit/Other	Title of Procedure	Rating Below (B) Meets (M) Exceeds (E) Expectations	Initial of Faculty and Date	Feedback Received Initial of Learner

ACADEMIC PRESENTATIONS

Date	Type Journal Club/Seminar/Clinical Case/Audit/Other	Title of Procedure	Rating Below (B) Meets (M) Exceeds (E) Expectations	Initial of Faculty and Date	Feedback Received Initial of Learner

SPECIAL ACHIEVEMENTS

Date	Type Presentation in Conference/Poster in Conference/Publication	Title of Procedure/Award	Name of Conference or Journal/Awarding Agency	Initial of Faculty and Date	Feedback Received Initial of Learner

SPECIAL ACHIEVEMENTS

Date	Type Presentation in Conference/ Poster in Conference/Publication	Title of Procedure	Name of Conference or Journal	Initial of Faculty and Date	Feedback Received Initial of Learner

SPECIAL TRAININGS/WORKSHOPS

Date	Workshop Theme	Organised by	Venue	Initial of Faculty and Date	Feedback Received Initial of Learner

SPECIAL TRAININGS/WORKSHOPS

Date	Workshop Theme	Organised by	Venue	Initial of Faculty and Date	Feedback Received Initial of Learner

SUGGESTED ACTIVITIES BY SURGICAL STUDENT (MBBS)

Sl. No.	Activity in Ward	Must know (M)/Good to know (G)
1.	Case record (history, progress notes, operative notes)	M
2.	Taking informed consent	M
3.	Follow up report (progress note)	M
4.	Preparing discharge summary	M
5.	Peripheral venous sample collection and transport	M
6.	Central venous sample collection	M
7.	Peripheral arterial sample collection and transport	M
8.	Intravenous cannula insertion	M
9.	Venesection/venous cut open/central line placement	M
10.	Resuscitation of critical patients	M
11.	Urinary catheterization (male)	M
12.	Urinary catheterization (female)	M
13.	Basic wound care (I)	M
14.	Basic bandaging (I)	M
15.	Wound dressings and application of splints	M
16.	Diabetic foot dressing	M
17.	Stoma care: change and dressing	M
18.	Wound suture (simple interrupted)	M
19.	Wound suture (mattress interrupted)	M
20.	Wound suture (blanket: continuous/horizontal mattress)	M
21.	Wound suture (subcuticular)	G
22.	Tracheostomy and endotracheal intubation	G
23.	Involvement in treatment planning and administration	M
24.	Monitoring of vitals (routine)-TPR-BP	M
25.	Monitoring of vitals (sick)-TPR-BP	M
26.	Input/output charting/monitoring	M
27.	Intravenous fluid (order)/monitoring to avoid overload	M
28.	Central venous pressure monitoring (observation)	M
29.	Blood transfusion	M
30.	Abdominal girth charting	M
31.	Resuscitation (ABC)	M
32.	Management of person in shock	M
33.	Management of person in coma	M
34.	Prevention of pressure sore	M
35.	Receiving of immediate post-operative patient	M
36.	Should be able to demonstrate understanding of World Health Organisation cause of death reporting and data quality requirements	M
37.	Should be able to demonstrate understanding of the use of national and state/local cause of death statistics	M
38.	Advise about prognosis of acute and chronic surgical illnesses, head injury, trauma, burns and cancer. Counsel patients regarding the same	M
39.	Advise about rehabilitation of patients after surgery and assist them for early recovery	M

Sl. No.	Activity in Operation Theatre (Minor/Major)	Must know (M)/Good to know (G)
1.	Circumcision	G
2.	Reduction of paraphimosis/dorsal slit	G
3.	Operation for hydrocele (Eversion/Lord's)	G
4.	Excision of swelling (lipoma/fibroma/fibroadenoma, etc.)	M
5.	Abscess drainage (perianal/breast/superficial abscess)	M
6.	Wound debridement	M
7.	Assisting major operative procedure	G
8.	Basic suturing (I)	M
9.	Performing FNAC	M
10.	Biopsy of surface tumours/lymph node/trucut	M
11.	Vasectomy (non-scalpel)	G
12.	Catheterization of patients with acute retention or trocar cystostomy	M
13.	Assisting in laparoscopic/minimally invasive surgery	G
14.	Lymph node biopsy	G
15.	Basic surgical procedures for major and minor surgical illnesses	M